# RENAL DIET COOKBOOK FOR BEGINNER:

*200+ Delicious and Easy Recipes with
Low Sodium, Potassium and Phosphorus.
Includes A Carefully Selected 21-Days Meal Plan
to Avoid Dialysis*

# © Copyright 2020 - All rights reserved.

The content contained within this book may not be reproduced, duplicated or transmitted without direct written permission from the author or the publisher.

Under no circumstances will any blame or legal responsibility be held against the publisher, or author, for any damages, reparation, or monetary loss due to the information contained within this book. Either directly or indirectly.

## Legal Notice:

This book is copyright protected. This book is only for personal use. You cannot amend, distribute, sell, use, quote or paraphrase any part, or the content within this book, without the consent of the author or publisher.

## Disclaimer Notice:

Please note the information contained within this document is for educational and entertainment purposes only. All effort has been executed to present accurate, up to date, and reliable, complete information. No warranties of any kind are declared or implied. Readers acknowledge that the author is not engaging in the rendering of legal, financial, medical or professional advice. The content within this book has been derived from various sources. Please consult a licensed professional before attempting any techniques outlined in this book.

By reading this document, the reader agrees that under no circumstances is the author responsible for any losses, direct or indirect, which are incurred as a result of the use of information contained within this document, including, but not limited to, errors, omissions, or inaccuracies.

# Table of Contents

INTRODUCTION .................................................. 8
**CHAPTER 1: UNDERSTANDING KIDNEY DISEASE** ....... 10
    What Do the Kidneys Do? .............................. 10
    What Causes Kidney Disease? ....................... 10
    Treatment Plans for Chronic Kidney Disease (CKD) .... 11
**CHAPTER 2: THE CAUSES OF RENAL FAILURE** ............ 14
    Symptoms of kidney disease? ........................ 15
    Diagnose With Kidney Disease ....................... 15
**CHAPTER 3: WHAT YOU CAN EAT, WHAT TO AVOID** . 18
    Foods You Need ............................................. 18
    Foods you Need to Avoid ............................... 19
    Renal Diet Shopping List ................................ 20
**CHAPTER 4: MEAL PLAN** ........................................ 26
**CHAPTER 5: BREAKFAST** ........................................ 28
1. EASY TURNIP PUREE ........................................ 28
2. GREEN LETTUCE BACON BREAKFAST BAKE ......... 29
3. HEALTHY GREEN LETTUCE TOMATO MUFFINS ... 30
4. CHICKEN EGG BREAKFAST MUFFINS .................. 31
5. BREAKFAST EGG SALAD .................................... 32
6. VEGETABLE TOFU SCRAMBLE ............................ 33
7. CHEESE COCONUT PANCAKES ........................... 34
8. CHEESY SCRAMBLED EGGS WITH FRESH HERBS .. 35
9. COCONUT BREAKFAST SMOOTHIE ..................... 36
10. TURKEY AND GREEN LETTUCE SCRAMBLE ON MELBA TOAST ........................................................ 37
11. VEGETABLE OMELET ...................................... 38
12. MEXICAN STYLE BURRITOS ............................. 39
13. BULGUR, COUSCOUS AND BUCKWHEAT CEREAL 40
14. SWEET PANCAKES .......................................... 41
15. BREAKFAST SMOOTHIE ................................... 42
16. BUCKWHEAT AND GRAPEFRUIT PORRIDGE ....... 43
17. EGG AND VEGGIE MUFFINS ............................. 44
18. SALAD WITH VINAIGRETTE ............................. 45
19. SALAD WITH LEMON DRESSING ...................... 46
20. SHRIMP WITH SALSA ...................................... 47
21. PESTO PORK CHOPS ........................................ 48
22. TURKEY BURGERS .......................................... 49
**CHAPTER 6: LUNCH** ............................................. 50
23. DOLMAS WRAP .............................................. 50
24. SALAD AL TONNO ........................................... 51
25. ARLECCHINO RICE SALAD ............................... 52
26. SAUTEED CHICKPEA AND LENTIL MIX .............. 53
27. CRAZY JAPANESE POTATO AND BEEF CROQUETTES ........................................................ 54
28. TRADITIONAL BLACK BEAN CHILI .................... 55
29. GREEN PALAK PANEER ................................... 56
30. CUCUMBER SANDWICH .................................. 57
31. PIZZA PITAS ................................................... 58
32. LETTUCE WRAPS WITH CHICKEN .................... 59
33. TURKEY PINWHEELS ....................................... 60
34. CHICKEN TACOS ............................................. 61
35. TUNA TWIST .................................................. 62
36. CIABATTA ROLLS WITH CHICKEN PESTO .......... 63
37. MARINATED SHRIMP PASTA SALAD ................. 64
38. PEANUT BUTTER AND JELLY GRILLED SANDWICH ............................................................................ 65
39. GRILLED ONION AND PEPPER JACK GRILLED CHEESE SANDWICH ................................................ 66
40. CRISPY LEMON CHICKEN ................................ 67
41. MEXICAN STEAK TACOS .................................. 68
42. BEER PORK RIBS ............................................. 69
43. MEXICAN CHORIZO SAUSAGE ......................... 70
44. EGGPLANT CASSEROLE ................................... 71
45. PIZZA WITH CHICKEN AND PESTO ................... 72
46. SHRIMP QUESADILLA ..................................... 73
47. GRILLED CORN ON THE COB ........................... 74
48. COUSCOUS WITH VEGGIES .............................. 75
49. EASY EGG SALAD ............................................ 76
50. CAULIFLOWER RICE AND COCONUT ................ 77

| # | Recipe | Page |
|---|---|---|
| 51. | KALE AND GARLIC PLATTER | 78 |
| 52. | BLISTERED BEANS AND ALMOND | 79 |
| 53. | CUCUMBER SOUP | 80 |
| 54. | EGGPLANT SALAD | 81 |
| 55. | CAJUN CRAB | 82 |
| 56. | MUSHROOM PORK CHOPS | 83 |
| 57. | CARAMELIZED PORK CHOPS | 84 |
| 58. | MEDITERRANEAN PORK | 85 |
| 59. | GROUND BEEF AND BELL PEPPERS | 86 |
| 60. | SPICED UP PORK CHOPS | 87 |
| 61. | JUICY SALMON DISH | 88 |
| 62. | PLATTER-O-BRUSSELS | 89 |
| 63. | ALMOND CHICKEN | 90 |
| 64. | BLACKBERRY CHICKEN WINGS | 91 |
| 65. | AROMATIC CARROT CREAM | 92 |
| 66. | MUSHROOMS VELVET SOUP | 93 |
| 67. | EASY LETTUCE WRAPS | 94 |
| 68. | SPAGHETTI WITH PESTO | 95 |
| 69. | VEGETABLE CASSEROLE | 96 |
| 70. | APPETIZING RICE SALAD | 97 |
| 71. | SPICED WRAPS | 98 |
| 72. | RUMP ROAST | 99 |

**CHAPTER 7: DINNER ............................................. 100**

| # | Recipe | Page |
|---|---|---|
| 73. | BEEF KABOBS WITH PEPPER | 100 |
| 74. | ONE-POT BEEF ROAST | 101 |
| 75. | CABBAGE AND BEEF FRY | 102 |
| 76. | CALIFORNIA PORK CHOPS | 103 |
| 77. | CARIBBEAN TURKEY CURRY | 104 |
| 78. | CHICKEN FAJITAS | 105 |
| 79. | CHICKEN VERONIQUE | 106 |
| 80. | CHICKEN AND APPLE CURRY | 107 |
| 81. | LONDON BROIL | 108 |
| 82. | SIRLOIN WITH SQUASH AND PINEAPPLE | 109 |
| 83. | SLOW-COOKED BBQ BEEF | 110 |
| 84. | LEMON SPROUTS | 111 |
| 85. | LEMON AND BROCCOLI PLATTER | 112 |
| 86. | CHICKEN LIVER STEW | 113 |
| 87. | SIMPLE LAMB CHOPS | 114 |
| 88. | CHICKEN AND MUSHROOM STEW | 115 |
| 89. | ROASTED CARROT SOUP | 116 |
| 90. | GARLIC AND BUTTER-FLAVORED COD | 117 |
| 91. | TILAPIA BROCCOLI PLATTER | 118 |
| 92. | PARSLEY SCALLOPS | 119 |
| 93. | BLACKENED CHICKEN | 120 |
| 94. | SPICY PAPRIKA LAMB CHOPS | 121 |
| 95. | MUSHROOM AND OLIVE SIRLOIN STEAK | 122 |
| 96. | PARSLEY AND CHICKEN BREAST | 123 |
| 97. | SIMPLE MUSTARD CHICKEN | 124 |
| 98. | GOLDEN EGGPLANT FRIES | 125 |
| 99. | VERY WILD MUSHROOM PILAF | 126 |
| 100. | SPORTY BABY CARROTS | 127 |
| 101. | SAUCY GARLIC GREENS | 128 |
| 102. | GARDEN SALAD | 129 |
| 103. | SPICY CABBAGE DISH | 130 |
| 104. | EXTREME BALSAMIC CHICKEN | 131 |
| 105. | ENJOYABLE GREEN LETTUCE AND BEAN MEDLEY | 132 |
| 106. | TANTALIZING CAULIFLOWER AND DILL MASH | 133 |
| 107. | PEAS SOUP | 134 |
| 108. | MINTY LAMB STEW | 135 |
| 109. | SPICY MUSHROOM STIR-FRY | 136 |
| 110. | CURRIED VEGGIES AND RICE | 137 |
| 111. | SPICY VEGGIE PANCAKES | 138 |
| 112. | EGG AND VEGGIE FAJITAS | 139 |
| 113. | VEGETABLE BIRYANI | 140 |
| 114. | CREAMY TUNA SALAD | 141 |
| 115. | CREAMY MUSHROOM SOUP | 142 |
| 116. | PORK SOUP | 143 |
| 117. | THAI CHICKEN SOUP | 144 |
| 118. | TASTY PUMPKIN SOUP | 145 |

| # | Title | Page |
|---|---|---|
| 119. | EASY ZUCCHINI SOUP | 146 |
| 120. | QUICK TOMATO SOUP | 147 |
| 121. | SPICY CHICKEN SOUP | 148 |
| 122. | SHREDDED PORK SOUP | 149 |
| 123. | CREAMY CHICKEN GREEN LETTUCE SOUP | 150 |
| 124. | SHRIMP PAELLA | 151 |
| 125. | SALMON & PESTO SALAD | 152 |
| 126. | BAKED FENNEL & GARLIC SEA BASS | 153 |
| 127. | LEMON, GARLIC, CILANTRO TUNA AND RICE | 154 |
| 128. | COD & GREEN BEAN RISOTTO | 155 |
| 129. | SARDINE FISH CAKES | 156 |
| 130. | 4-INGREDIENTS SALMON FILLET | 157 |
| 131. | SPANISH COD IN SAUCE | 158 |
| 132. | SALMON BAKED IN FOIL WITH FRESH THYME | 159 |
| 133. | POACHED HALIBUT IN ORANGE SAUCE | 160 |

**CHAPTER 8: SNACK RECIPES ............................. 162**

| # | Title | Page |
|---|---|---|
| 134. | VEGGIE SNACK | 162 |
| 135. | HEALTHY SPICED NUTS | 163 |
| 136. | ROASTED ASPARAGUS | 164 |
| 137. | LOW-FAT MANGO SALSA | 165 |
| 138. | VINEGAR & SALT KALE | 166 |
| 139. | CARROT AND PARSNIPS FRENCH FRIES | 167 |
| 140. | APPLE & STRAWBERRY SNACK | 168 |
| 141. | CANDIED MACADAMIA NUTS | 169 |
| 142. | CINNAMON APPLE FRIES | 170 |
| 143. | LEMON POPS | 171 |
| 144. | EASY NO-BAKE COCONUT COOKIES | 172 |
| 145. | ROASTED CHILI-VINEGAR PEANUTS | 173 |
| 146. | POPCORN WITH SUGAR AND SPICE | 174 |
| 147. | EGGPLANT AND CHICKPEA BITES | 175 |
| 148. | BABA GHANOUJ | 176 |
| 149. | BAKED PITA FRIES | 177 |
| 150. | HERBAL CREAM CHEESE TARTINES | 178 |
| 151. | MIXES OF SNACKS | 179 |
| 152. | SPICY CRAB DIP | 180 |
| 153. | BAKED APPLES WITH CHERRIES AND WALNUTS | 181 |
| 154. | EASY PEACH CRUMBLE | 182 |

**CHAPTER 9: 40 RECIPES FOR THOSE WHO HAVE DIALYSIS: BREAKFAST ............................ 184**

| # | Title | Page |
|---|---|---|
| 155. | BREAKFAST SALAD FROM GRAINS AND FRUITS | 184 |
| 156. | FRENCH TOAST WITH APPLESAUCE | 185 |
| 157. | BAGELS MADE HEALTHY | 186 |
| 158. | CORNBREAD WITH SOUTHERN TWIST | 187 |
| 159. | GRANDMA'S PANCAKE SPECIAL | 188 |
| 160. | PASTA WITH INDIAN LENTILS | 189 |
| 161. | SHRIMP BRUSCHETTA | 190 |
| 162. | STRAWBERRY MUESLI | 191 |
| 163. | YOGURT BULGUR | 192 |
| 164. | MOZZARELLA CHEESE OMELET | 193 |

**CHAPTER 10: LUNCH ............................ 194**

| # | Title | Page |
|---|---|---|
| 165. | COUSCOUS AND SHERRY VINAIGRETTE | 194 |
| 166. | PERSIAN CHICKEN | 195 |
| 167. | RATATOUILLE | 196 |
| 168. | JICAMA NOODLES | 197 |
| 169. | CRACK SLAW | 198 |
| 170. | VEGAN CHILI | 199 |
| 171. | CHOW MEIN | 199 |
| 172. | MUSHROOM TACOS | 201 |
| 173. | LIME GREEN LETTUCE AND CHICKPEAS SALAD | 202 |
| 174. | FRIED RICE WITH KALE | 203 |
| 175. | STIR-FRIED GINGERY VEGGIES | 204 |

**CHAPTER 11: DINNER ............................ 206**

| # | Title | Page |
|---|---|---|
| 176. | FISH EN' PAPILLOTE | 206 |
| 177. | PESTO PASTA SALAD | 207 |
| 178. | BARLEY BLUEBERRY SALAD | 208 |
| 179. | PASTA WITH CREAMY BROCCOLI SAUCE | 209 |
| 180. | ASPARAGUS FRIED RICE | 210 |
| 181. | BEEF AND CHILI STEW | 211 |

| | | | | | |
|---|---|---|---|---|---|
| 182. | STICKY PULLED BEEF OPEN SANDWICHES .... 212 | | 192. | CHOCOLATE CHIA SEED PUDDING ............... 222 |
| 183. | HERBY BEEF STROGANOFF AND FLUFFY RICE ............................................................................ 213 | | 193. | CHOCOLATE-MINT TRUFFLES ....................... 223 |
| 184. | CHUNKY BEEF AND POTATO SLOW ROAST .. 214 | | 194. | PERSONAL MANGO PIES .............................. 224 |
| 185. | SPICED LAMB BURGERS ................................ 215 | | 195. | GRILLED PEACH SUNDAES ............................ 225 |
| 186. | PORK LOINS WITH LEEKS .............................. 216 | | 196. | BLUEBERRY SWIRL CAKE .............................. 226 |
| 187. | THE KALE AND GREEN LETTUCE SOUP ......... 217 | | 197. | PEANUT BUTTER COOKIES ............................ 227 |
| 188. | JAPANESE ONION SOUP ............................... 218 | | 198. | DELICIOUSLY GOOD SCONES ....................... 228 |
| 189. | AMAZING BROCCOLI AND CAULIFLOWER SOUP ............................................................................ 219 | | 199. | MIXED BERRY COBBLER ................................ 229 |

**CHAPTER 12: SNACKS ................................................. 220**

| | | | | | |
|---|---|---|---|---|---|
| | | | 200. | BLUEBERRY ESPRESSO BROWNIES ............... 230 |
| 190. | LEMON THINS ............................................... 220 | | 201. | COFFEE BROWNIES ....................................... 231 |
| 191. | SNICKERDOODLE CHICKPEA BLONDIES ........ 221 | | | |

**CONCLUSION ............................................................. 232**

# Introduction

The renal diet is a diet for people (mostly diabetics, CKD patients and chronic kidney disease patients) who have special needs when it comes to their nutritional intake. Mostly it includes high amounts of proteins, sodium, potassium, calcium, phosphorus and low amounts of phosphorus, sodium, potassium, potassium, proteins, fat and proteins, so that it usually limits the fat content of food and sets the protein to carbohydrate ratio quite high as well.

A low sodium renal diet can be achieved by adding potassium, low sodium intake, and adding fiber. Many people struggle with adding extra fiber to the diet, and many times it is treated as an unhealthy factor. But when added to the renal diet, you will soon understand the benefits.

Phosphate: Consumption of phosphate becomes dangerous when kidney failure reaches 80% and goes to the 4th/5th stage of kidney failure. So, it is better to lower your phosphate intake by counting the calories and minerals.

Potassium: After getting diagnosed, if your results show your potassium level is high in the blood, then you should restrict your potassium intake. Baked and fried potatoes are very high in potassium. Leafy greens, fruit juices are high in potassium. You can still enjoy vegetables that are low in potassium.

Sodium: Adding salt is very important in our food, but when you are suffering from kidney problems, you have to omit or minimize your salt intake. Too much sodium intake can trigger high blood pressure and fluid retention in the body. You need to find substitutes that help season your food. Herbs and spices that are extracted from plants are a good option. Using garlic, pepper, mustard can increase the taste of your food without adding any salt. Avoid artificial "salts" that are low in sodium because they are high in potassium, which is also dangerous for kidney health.

Recipes from this cookbook are simple, delicious, and healthy. You can even use them as an inspiration to experiment and create your renal diet recipes. These samples can also be considered as snacks for you throughout the day.

Below is a list of food/nutrients you should avoid preventing kidney-related problems: Food to avoid Limit/Avoid Alcohol No more than two drinks a day According to The Association of Diabetic Retinopathy, dialysis and kidney transplantation, Alcohol can be safe if consumed in moderation. 1-2 alcoholic beverages a day while dieting is acceptable. Alcohol consumption should be avoided completely if this is unattainable. Milk and milk products No more than two glasses a day As per " The American Heart Association, " milk and milk products including cheese, cheese products and yogurt can be allowed without any accommodations. However, it is recommended to replace them with low-fat dairy products. Vegetables and beans No more than 2 cups a day, except for one serving a day of soy milk or other protein-rich beverages. A kidney diet is not complete without vegetables and beans. " United States National Library of Medicine" specifies that one banana, one apple, a serving of broccoli, and one cup of tomato juice can be substituted with protein-rich food. Grains No more than two servings a day. It is recommended to substitute them with another high protein low-fat food regular, such as poultry or fish. A cup of milk and two saltine crackers are also allowed a day.

If you're already used to the renal diet, you can work with the recipes from this cookbook. You can use the guide for more severe and careful renal diet beginners. If you want to live a happy, healthy renal diet, try these simple recipes for a better taste!

# CHAPTER 1:

# Understanding Kidney Disease

Kidney disease is becoming more prevalent in the United States, and so we need to learn as much about it as we can. The more we educate ourselves, the more we can do to take care of this important bodily system. If you've been diagnosed with chronic kidney disease (CKD), education can empower you to most effectively and purposefully manage the disease. Once you have a full understanding of what chronic kidney disease is, you can begin to take charge of your evolving health needs. Making healthy changes early in the stages of kidney disease will help determine how well you will manage your kidney health. I am here to guide you, every step of the way. Like any new process, it may seem intimidating at first. But this chapter provides the foundation for learning and will help you understand kidney disease as you begin your journey to healthier kidneys.

## What Do the Kidneys Do?

Our kidneys are small, but they do powerful things to keep our bodies in balance. They are bean-shaped, about the size of a fist, and are located in the middle of the back, on the left and right sides of the spine, just below the rib cage. When everything is working properly, the kidneys do many important jobs such as:

- Filter waste materials from the blood
- Remove extra fluid, or water, from the body
- Release hormones that help manage blood pressure
- Stimulate bone marrow to make red blood cells
- Make an active form of vitamin D that promotes strong, healthy bones

## What Causes Kidney Disease?

There are many causes of kidney disease, including physical injury or disorders that can damage the kidneys, but the two leading causes of kidney disease are diabetes and high blood pressure. These underlying conditions also put people at risk for developing cardiovascular disease. Early treatment may not only slow down the progression of the disease, but also reduce your risk of developing heart disease or stroke.

Kidney disease can affect anyone, at any age. African Americans, Hispanics, and American Indians are at increased risk for kidney failure, because these groups have a greater prevalence of diabetes and high blood pressure.

When we digest protein, our bodies create waste products. As blood flows through the capillaries, the waste products are filtered through the urine. Substances such as protein and red blood cells are too big to pass through the capillaries and so stay in the blood. All the extra work takes a toll on the kidneys. When kidney disease is detected in the early stages, several treatments may prevent the worsening of the disease. If kidney disease is detected in the later stages, high amounts of protein in your urine, called macroalbuminuria, can lead to end-stage renal disease.

The second leading cause of kidney disease is high blood pressure, also known as hypertension. One in three Americans is at risk for kidney disease because of hypertension. Although there is no cure for hypertension, certain medications, a low-sodium diet, and physical activity can lower blood pressure.

The kidneys help manage blood pressure, but when blood pressure is high, the heart has to work overtime at pumping blood. When the force of blood flow is high, blood vessels start to stretch so the blood can flow more easily. The stretching and scarring weaken the blood vessels throughout the entire body, including the kidneys. And when the kidneys' blood vessels are injured, they may not remove the waste and extra fluid from the body, creating a dangerous cycle, because the extra fluid in the blood vessels can increase blood pressure even more.

With diabetes, excess blood sugar remains in the bloodstream. The high blood sugar levels can damage the blood vessels in the kidneys and elsewhere in the body. And since high blood pressure is a complication from diabetes, the extra pressure can weaken the walls of the blood vessels, which can lead to a heart attack or stroke.

Other conditions, such as drug abuse and certain autoimmune diseases, can also cause injury to the kidneys. In fact, every drug we put into our body has to pass through the kidneys for filtration.

An autoimmune disease is one in which the immune system, designed to protect the body from illness, sees the body as an invader and attacks its own systems, including the kidneys. Some forms of lupus, for example, attack the kidneys. Another autoimmune disease that can lead to kidney failure is Good pasture syndrome, a group of conditions that affect the kidneys and the lungs. The damage to the kidneys from autoimmune diseases can lead to chronic kidney disease and kidney failure.

## Treatment Plans for Chronic Kidney Disease (CKD)

The best way to manage CKD is to be an active participant in your treatment program, regardless of your stage of renal disease. Proper treatment involves a combination of working with a healthcare team, adhering to a renal diet, and making healthy lifestyle decisions. These can all have a profoundly positive effect on your kidney disease—especially watching how you eat.

Working with your healthcare team. When you have kidney disease, working in partnership with your healthcare team can be extremely important in your treatment program as well as being personally empowering. Regularly meeting with your physician or healthcare team can arm you with resources and information that help you make informed decisions regarding your treatment needs, and provide you with a much-needed opportunity to vent, share information, get advice, and receive support in effectively managing this illness.

Adhering to a renal diet. The heart of this book is the renal diet. Sticking to this diet can make a huge difference in your health and vitality. Like any change, following the diet may not be easy at first. Important changes to your diet, particularly early on, can possibly prevent the need for dialysis. These changes include limiting salt, eating a low-protein diet, reducing fat intake, and getting enough calories if you need to lose weight. Be honest with yourself first and foremost—learn what you need, and consider your personal goals and obstacles. Start by making small changes. It is okay to have some slip-ups—we all do. With guidance and support, these small changes will become habits of your promising new lifestyle. In no time, you will begin taking control of your diet and health.

Making healthy lifestyle decisions. Lifestyle choices play a crucial part in our health, especially when it comes to helping regulate kidney disease. Lifestyle choices such as allotting time for physical activity, getting enough sleep, managing weight, reducing stress, and limiting smoking and alcohol will help you take control of your overall health, making it easier to manage your kidney disease. Follow this simple formula: Keep toxins out of your body as much as you can, and build up your immune system with a good balance of exercise, relaxation, and sleep.

# CHAPTER 2:

# The Causes of Renal Failure

Renal disease, according to experts, requires early diagnosis and targeted treatment to prevent or delay both a condition of acute or chronic renal failure and the appearance of cardiovascular complications to which it is often associated.

In fact, hypertension and diabetes, not adequately controlled by drug therapy, prostatic hypertrophy, kidney stones or bulky tumors can promote onset as they reduce the normal flow of urine, increase the pressure inside the kidneys and limit functionality.

Or the kidney damage can be determined by inflammatory processes (pyelonephritis, glomerulonephritis) or by the formation of cysts inside the kidneys (polycystic kidney disease) or by the chronic use of some drugs, alcohol and drugs consumed in excess.

A fundamental role in alleviating the work of the already compromised kidneys is carried out by the diet which is, therefore, the first prevention. It must be studied with an expert nutritionist or a nephrologist in order to maintain or reach an ideal weight on the one hand and on the other to reduce the intake of sodium (salt), and the consequent control of blood pressure, and / or other substances (minerals), without creating malnutrition or nutritional deficiencies. Particular attention should also be paid to cholesterol, triglycerides and blood sugar levels.

Understanding what causes kidney failure goes a long way to deciding just what kind of treatment you should focus on. The most important factor that you should focus on is, of course, your diet. But as you focus on your diet, make sure that you are following your doctor's instructions, in the event of other complications. Let us look at a few of the common causes of kidney diseases.

## Diabetes

We do know that diabetes is one of the leading causes of CKD. But we have yet to understand in detail why and how it can cause so much harm to the kidneys.

Time for a crash course in diabetes. What many may already know is that diabetes affects our body's insulin production rate. But what many may not know is the extent of damage that diabetes can cause to the kidneys.

## High Blood Pressure

An important thing to remember here is that high blood pressure can be both a cause and symptom of CKD, similar to the case of diabetes.

So, what exactly is blood pressure? People often throw the term around, but they are unable to pinpoint exactly what happens when the pressure in the blood increases.

## Autoimmune Diseases

IgA nephropathy and lupus are two examples of autoimmune diseases that can lead to kidney diseases. But just what exactly are autoimmune diseases?

They are conditions where your immune system perceives your body as a threat and begins to attack it.

We all know that the immune system is like the defense force of our body. It is responsible for guiding the soldiers of our body, known as white blood cells, or WBCs. The immune system is responsible for fighting against foreign materials, such as viruses and bacteria. When the system senses these foreign bodies, various fighter cells, including the WBCs, are deployed in order to combat the threat.

Typically, your immune system is a self-learning system. This means that it is capable of understanding the threat and memorizing its features, behaviors, and attack patterns. This is an important capability of the immune system since it allows the system to differentiate between our own cells and foreign cells. But when you have an autoimmune disease, your immune system suddenly considers certain parts of your body, such as your skin or joints, as foreign. It then proceeds to create antibodies that begin to

## Symptoms of kidney disease?

If kidney disease progresses, then the blood level of end products of metabolism increases; this in turn, is the cause of feeling unwell. Various health problems may occur, such as high blood pressure, anemia (anemia), bone disease, premature cardiovascular calcification, discoloration, and change in the composition and volume of urine.

As the disease progresses, the main symptoms can be:
- Weakness, a feeling of weakness
- Trouble sleeping
- Lack of appetite
- Dry skin, itchy skin
- Muscle cramps especially at night
- Swelling in the legs
- Swelling around the eyes, especially in the morning

## Diagnose With Kidney Disease

There are two simple tests that your family doctor can prescribe to diagnose kidney disease.

Blood test: glomerular filtration rate (GFR) and serum creatinine level. Creatinine is one of those end products of protein metabolism, the level of which in the blood depends on age, gender, muscle mass, nutrition, physical activity, the foods taken before taking the sample (for example, a lot of meat was eaten), and some drugs. Creatinine is removed from the body through the kidneys, and if the work of the kidneys slows down, the level of creatinine in the blood plasma increases. Determining the level of creatinine alone is not sufficient for the diagnosis of chronic kidney disease since its value begins to exceed the upper limit of the norm only when GFR is decreased by half. GFR is calculated using a formula that includes four parameters which are; the creatinine reading, age, gender, and race of the patient. GFR shows the level at which the kidneys can filter. In the case of chronic kidney disease, the GFR indicator indicates the stage of the severity of kidney disease.

Urine analysis: the content of albumin in the urine is determined; also, the values of albumin and creatinine in the urine are determined by each other. Albumin is a protein in the urine that usually enters the urine in minimal quantities. Even a small increase in the level of albumin in the urine in some people may be an early sign of incipient kidney disease, especially in those with diabetes and high blood pressure. In the case of normal kidney function, albumin in the urine should not be more than 3 mg/mmol (or 30 mg/g). If albumin excretion increases even more, then it already speaks of kidney disease.

# CHAPTER 3:

# What you can Eat, What to Avoid

## Foods You Need

There are many foods that work well within the renal diet, and once you see the available variety, it will not seem as restrictive or difficult to follow. The key is focusing on the foods with a high level of nutrients, which make it easier for the kidneys to process waste by not adding too much that the body needs to discard. Balance is a major factor in maintaining and improving long-term renal function.

Garlic

Excellent, vitamin-rich food for the immune system, garlic is a tasty substitute for salt in a variety of dishes. It acts as a significant source of vitamin C and B6, while aiding the kidneys in ridding the body of unwanted toxins. It's a great, healthy way to add flavor to skillet meals, pasta, soups, and stews.

Berries

All berries are considered a good renal diet food due to their high level of fiber, antioxidants, and delicious taste, making them an easy option to include as a light snack or as an ingredient in smoothies, salads, and light desserts. Just one handful of blueberries can provide almost one day's vitamin C requirement, as well as a boost of fiber, which is good for weight loss and maintenance.

Bell Peppers

Flavorful and easy to enjoy both raw and cooked, bell peppers offer a good source of vitamin C, vitamin A, and fiber. Along with other kidney-friendly foods, they make the detoxification process much easier while boosting your body's nutrient level to prevent further health conditions and reduce existing deficiencies.

Onions

This nutritious and tasty vegetable is excellent as a companion to garlic in many dishes, or on its own. Like garlic, onions can provide flavor as an alternative to salt, and provides a good source of vitamin C, vitamin B, manganese, and fiber, as well. Adding just one quarter or half an onion is often enough for most meals, because of its strong, pungent flavor.

Macadamia Nuts

If you enjoy nuts and seeds as snacks, you may soon learn that many contain high amounts of phosphorus and should be avoided or limited as much as possible. Fortunately, macadamia nuts are an easier option to digest and process, as they contain much lower amounts of phosphorus and make an excellent substitute for other nuts. They are a good source of other nutrients, as well, such as vitamin B, copper, manganese, iron, and healthy fats.

Pineapple

Unlike other fruits that are high in potassium, pineapple is an option that can be enjoyed more often than bananas and kiwis. Citrus fruits are generally high in potassium as well, so if you find yourself craving an orange or grapefruit, choose pineapple instead. In addition to providing high levels of vitamin B and fiber, pineapples can reduce inflammation thanks to an enzyme called bromelain.

Mushrooms

In general, mushrooms are a safe, healthy option for the renal diet, especially the shiitake variety, which are high in nutrients such as selenium, vitamin B, and manganese. They contain a moderate amount of plant-based protein, which is easier for your body to digest and use than animal proteins. Shiitake and Portobello mushrooms are often used in vegan diets as a meat substitute, due to their texture and pleasant flavor.

## Foods you Need to Avoid

Eating restrictions might be different depending upon your level of kidney disease. If you are in the early stages of kidney disease, you may have different restrictions as compared to those who are at the end-stage renal disease, or kidney failure. In contrast to this, people with an end-stage renal disease requiring dialysis will face different eating restrictions. Let's discuss some of the foods to avoid while being on the renal diet.

Dark-Colored Colas contain calories, sugar, phosphorus, etc. They contain phosphorus to enhance flavor, increase its life and avoid discoloration. Which can be found in a product's ingredient list. This addition of phosphorus varies depending on the type of cola. Mostly, the dark-colored colas contain 50–100 mg in a 200-ml serving. Therefore, dark colas should be avoided on a renal diet.

Canned Foods including soups, vegetables, and beans, are low in cost but contain high amounts of sodium due to the addition of salt to increase its life. Due to this amount of sodium inclusion in canned goods, it is better that people with kidney disease should avoid consumption. Opt for lower-sodium content with the label "no salt added". One more way is to drain or rinse canned foods, such as canned beans and tuna, which could decrease the sodium content by 33–80%, depending on the product.

Brown Rice is a whole grain containing a higher concentration of potassium and phosphorus than its white rice counterpart. One cup of already cooked brown rice possesses about 150 mg of phosphorus and 154 mg of potassium, whereas, one cup of already cooked white rice has an amount of about 69 mg of phosphorus and 54 mg of potassium. Bulgur, buckwheat, pearled barley and couscous are equally beneficial, low-phosphorus options and might be a good alternative instead of brown rice.

Bananas are high potassium content, low in sodium, and provides 422 mg of potassium per banana. It might disturb your daily balanced potassium intake to 2,000 mg if a banana is a daily staple.

Whole-Wheat Bread may harm individuals with kidney disease. But for healthy individuals, it is recommended over refined, white flour bread. White bread is recommended instead of whole-wheat varieties for individuals with kidney disease just because it has phosphorus and potassium. If you add more bran and whole grains to the bread, then the amount of phosphorus and potassium contents goes higher.

Oranges and Orange Juice are enriched with vitamin C content and potassium. 184 grams provides 333 mg of potassium and 473 mg of potassium in one cup of orange juice. With these calculations, oranges and orange juice must be avoided or used in a limited amount while being on a renal diet.

Some of the high-potassium foods, likewise potatoes and sweet potatoes, could also be soaked or leached to lessen the concentration of potassium contents. Cut them into small and thin pieces and boil those for at least 10 minutes can reduce the potassium content by about 50%. Potatoes that are soaked in a wide pot of water for as low as four hours before cooking could possess even less potassium content than those not soaked before cooking. This is known as "potassium leaching," or the "double cook Direction."

If you are suffering from or living with kidney disease, reducing your potassium, phosphorus and sodium intake is an essential aspect of managing and tackling the disease. The foods with high-potassium, high-sodium, and high-phosphorus content listed above should always be limited or avoided. These restrictions and nutrients intakes may differ depending on the level of damage to your kidneys. Following a renal diet might be a daunting procedure and a restrictive one most of the time. But, working with your physician and nutrition specialist and a renal dietitian can assist you in formulating a renal diet specific to your individual needs.

## Renal Diet Shopping List

Vegetables:
- Arugula (raw)
- Alfalfa sprouts
- Bamboo shoots
- Asparagus
- Beans - pinto, wax, fava, green
- Bean sprouts
- Bitter melon (balsam pear)
- Broccoli
- Broad beans (boiled, fresh)
- Cactus
- Cabbage - red, swamp, Napa/ Suey Choy, skunk
- Carrots
- Calabash
- Celery
- Cauliflower
- Chayote
- Celeriac (cooked)
- Collard greens

- Chicory
- Cucumber
- Corn
- Okra
- Onions
- Pepitas
- (Green) Peas
- Peppers
- Radish
- Radicchio
- Seaweed
- Rapini (raw)
- Shallots
- Green lettuce (raw)
- Snow peas
- Dandelion greens (raw)
- Daikon
- Plant Leaves
- Drumstick
- Endive
- Eggplant
- Fennel bulb
- Escarole
- Fiddlehead greens
- Ferns
- Hearts of Palm
- Irish moss
- Hominy
- Jicama, raw
- Leeks
- Kale (raw)
- Mushrooms (raw white)
- Lettuce (raw)
- Mustard greens
- Squash
- Turnip

- Tomatillos (raw)
- Watercress
- Turnip greens
- Wax beans
- Water chestnuts (canned)
- Winter melon
- Wax gourd
- Zucchini (raw)

Fruits:
- Acerola Cherries
- Apple
- Blackberries
- Asian Pear
- Boysenberries
- Blueberries
- Cherries
- Casaba melon
- Clementine
- Chokeberries
- Crabapples
- Cloudberries
- Cranberries (fresh)
- Grapefruit
- Gooseberries
- Pomegranate
- Grapes
- Rambutan
- Quince
- Rhubarb
- Raspberries (fresh or frozen)
- Jujubes
- Golden Berry
- Kumquat
- Jackfruit
- Lingonberries
- Lemon

- Loganberries
- Lime
- Lychees
- Mango
- Mandarin orange
- Peach
- Pineapple
- Pear
- Plum
- Strawberries
- Rose-apple
- Tangerine
- Tangelo
- Watermelon

Fresh Meat, Seafood, and Poultry:

- Chicken
- Beef and Ground Beef
- Goat
- Duck
- Wild Game
- Pork
- Lamb
- Veal
- Turkey
- Fish

Milk, Eggs, and Dairy: Milk:

- Milk (½-1 cup/day)

Non-Dairy Milk:

- Almond Fresh (Original, Unsweetened, Vanilla)
- Almond Breeze (Original, Vanilla, Vanilla Unsweetened, Original Unsweetened)
- Silk True Almond Beverage (Unsweetened Original, Original, Vanilla, Unsweetened Vanilla)
- Good Karma Flax Delight (Vanilla, Original, Unsweetened)
- Rice Dream Rice Drink (Vanilla Classic, Non-Enriched Original Classic)
- Silk Soy Beverage (Original, Vanilla, Unsweetened)
- Natura Organic Fortified Rice Beverage (Original, Vanilla)
- PC Organics Fortified Rice Beverage

Other Dairy Products:
- Non-Hydrogenated Margarine (Salt-Free or Regular)
- Butter (Unsalted or Regular)
- Whipping Cream
- Sour Cream
- Whipped Cream

# CHAPTER 4:

# Meal Plan

| Days | Breakfast | Lunch | Dinner |
|---|---|---|---|
| 1 | Breakfast Salad from Grains and Fruits | Dolmas Wrap | Beef Kabobs with Pepper |
| 2 | French toast with Applesauce | Salad al Tonno | One-Pot Beef Roast |
| 3 | Bagels Made Healthy | Arlecchino Rice Salad | Cabbage and Beef Fry |
| 4 | Cornbread with Southern Twist | Sauteed Chickpea and Lentil Mix | California Pork Chops |
| 5 | Grandma's Pancake Special | Crazy Japanese Potato and Beef Croquettes | Caribbean Turkey Curry |
| 6 | Pasta with Indian Lentils | Traditional Black Bean Chili | Chicken Fajitas |
| 7 | Shrimp Bruschetta | Green Palak Paneer | Chicken Veronique |
| 8 | Strawberry Muesli | Cucumber Sandwich | Chicken and Apple Curry |
| 9 | Yogurt Bulgur | Pizza Pitas | London Broil |
| 10 | Mozzarella Cheese Omelet | Lettuce Wraps with Chicken | Sirloin with Squash and Pineapple |
| 11 | Coconut Breakfast Smoothie | Turkey Pinwheels | Slow-Cooked BBQ Beef |
| 12 | Easy Turnip Puree | Chicken Tacos | Lemon Sprouts |
| 13 | Green lettuce Bacon Breakfast Bake | Tuna Twist | Lemon and Broccoli Platter |
| 14 | Healthy Green lettuce Tomato Muffins | Ciabatta Rolls with Chicken Pesto | Chicken Liver Stew |
| 15 | Chicken Egg Breakfast Muffins | Marinated Shrimp Pasta Salad | Simple Lamb Chops |
| 16 | Breakfast Egg Salad | Peanut Butter and Jelly Grilled Sandwich | Chicken and Mushroom Stew |

| 17 | Vegetable Tofu Scramble | Grilled Onion and Pepper Jack Grilled Cheese Sandwich | Roasted Carrot Soup |
|---|---|---|---|
| 18 | Cheese Coconut Pancakes | Crispy Lemon Chicken | Garlic and Butter-Flavored Cod |
| 19 | Cheesy Scrambled Eggs with Fresh Herbs | Mexican Steak Tacos | Tilapia Broccoli Platter |
| 20 | Coconut Breakfast Smoothie | Beer Pork Ribs | Parsley Scallops |
| 21 | Turkey and Green lettuce Scramble on Melba Toast | Mexican Chorizo Sausage | Blackened Chicken |

# CHAPTER 5:

# Breakfast

## 1. Easy Turnip Puree

**Preparation Time:** 10 minutes

**Cooking Time:** 12 minutes

**Servings:** 4

**Ingredients:**

- 1 1/2 lbs. turnips, peeled and chopped
- 1 tsp. dill
- 3 bacon slices, cooked and chopped
- 2 tbsp. fresh chives, chopped

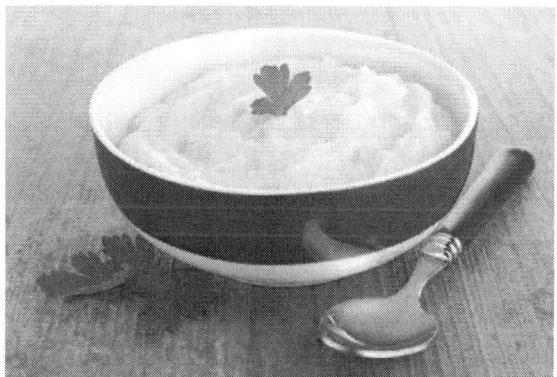

**Directions:**

1. Add turnip into the boiling water and cook for 12 minutes. Drain well and place in a food processor.
2. Add dill and process until smooth.
3. Transfer turnip puree into the bowl and top with bacon and chives.
4. Serve and enjoy.

**Nutrition:**

Calories 127

Fat 6g

Carbohydrates 11.6g

Sugar 7g

Protein 6.8g

Cholesterol 16 mg

## 2. Green lettuce Bacon Breakfast Bake

**Preparation Time:** 10 minutes

**Cooking Time:** 45 minutes

**Servings:** 6

**Ingredients:**

- 10 eggs
- 3 cups baby green lettuce, chopped
- 1 tbsp. olive oil
- 8 bacon slices, cooked and chopped
- 2 Red bell peppers, sliced
- 2 tbsp. chives, chopped
- Pepper
- Salt

**Directions:**

1. Preheat the oven to 350 F.
2. Spray a baking dish with cooking spray and set aside.
3. Heat oil in a pan
4. Add green lettuce and cook until green lettuce wilted.
5. In a mixing bowl, whisk eggs and salt. Add green lettuce and chives and stir well.
6. Pour egg mixture into the baking dish.
7. Top with Red bell peppers and bacon and bake for 45 minutes.
8. Serve and enjoy.

**Nutrition:**

Calories 273

Fat 20.4g

Carbohydrates 3.1g

Sugar 1.7g

Protein 19.4g

Cholesterol 301 mg

## 3. Healthy Green lettuce Tomato Muffins

**Preparation Time:** 10 minutes

**Cooking Time:** 20 minutes

**Servings:** 12

**Ingredients:**

- 12 eggs
- 1/2 tsp. Italian seasoning
- 1 cup Red bell peppers, chopped
- 4 tbsp. water
- 1 cup fresh green lettuce, chopped
- Pepper
- Salt

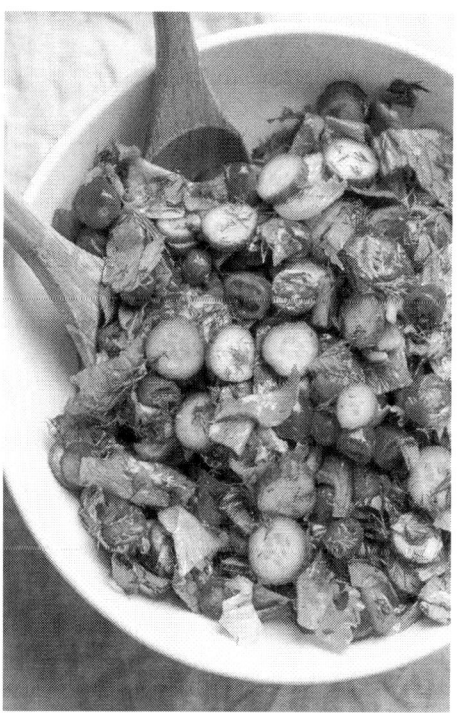

**Directions:**

1. Preheat the oven to 350 F. Spray a muffin tray with cooking spray and set aside.
2. In a mixing bowl, whisk eggs with water, Italian seasoning, pepper, and salt.
3. Add green lettuce and Red bell peppers and stir well.
4. Pour egg mixture into the prepared muffin tray and bake for 20 minutes.
5. Serve and enjoy.

**Nutrition:**

Calories 67

Fat 4.5g

Carbohydrates 1g

Sugar 0.8g

Protein 5.7g

Cholesterol 164 mg

## 4. Chicken Egg Breakfast Muffins

**Preparation Time:** 10 minutes

**Cooking Time:** 15 minutes

**Servings:** 12

**Ingredients:**

- 10 eggs
- 1 cup cooked chicken, chopped
- 3 tbsp. green onions, chopped
- 1/4 tsp. garlic powder
- Pepper
- Salt

**Directions:**

1. Preheat the oven to 400 F.
2. Spray a muffin tray with cooking spray and set aside.
3. In a large bowl, whisk eggs with garlic powder, pepper, and salt.
4. Add remaining ingredients and stir well.
5. Pour egg mixture into the muffin tray and bake for 15 minutes.
6. Serve and enjoy.

**Nutrition:**

Calories 71

Fat 4 g

Carbohydrates 0.4g

Sugar 0.3g

Protein 8g

Cholesterol 145 mg

## 5. Breakfast Egg Salad

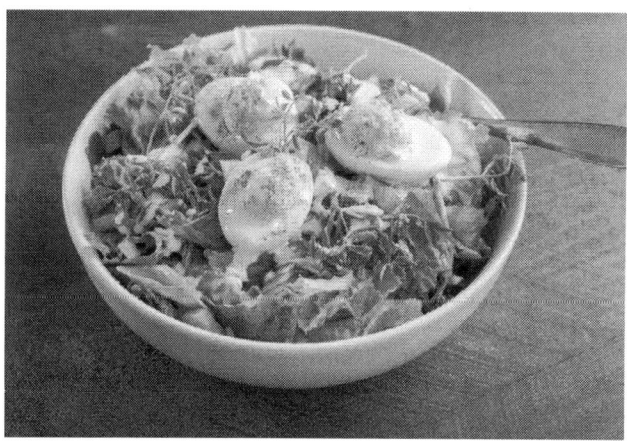

**Preparation Time:** 10 minutes

**Cooking Time:** 5 minutes

**Servings:** 4

**Ingredients:**

- 6 eggs, hard-boiled, peeled and chopped
- 1 tbsp. fresh dill, chopped
- 4 tbsp. mayonnaise
- Pepper
- Salt

**Directions:**

1. Add all ingredients into the large bowl and stir to mix. Serve and enjoy.

**Nutrition:**

Calories 140

Fat 10g

Carbohydrates 4g

Sugar 1g

Protein 8g

Cholesterol 245 mg

## 6. Vegetable Tofu Scramble

**Preparation Time:** 10 minutes

**Cooking Time:** 7 minutes

**Servings:** 2

**Ingredients:**

- 1/2 block firm tofu, crumbled
- 1/4 tsp. ground cumin
- 1 tbsp. turmeric
- 1 cup green lettuce
- 1/4 cup zucchini, chopped
- 1 tbsp. olive oil
- 1 tomato, chopped
- 1 tbsp. chives, chopped
- 1 tbsp. coriander, chopped
- Pepper
- Salt

**Directions:**

2. Heat oil in a pan over medium heat
3. Add tomato, zucchini, and green lettuce and sauté for 2 minutes.
4. Add tofu, cumin, turmeric, pepper, and salt and sauté for 5 minutes.
5. Top with chives, and coriander.
6. Serve and enjoy.

**Nutrition:**

Calories 101

Fat 8.5 g

Carbohydrates 5.1g

Sugar 1.4g

Protein 3.1g

Cholesterol 0 mg

## 7. Cheese Coconut Pancakes

**Preparation Time:** 10 minutes

**Cooking Time:** 5 minutes

**Servings:** 1

**Ingredients:**

- 2 eggs
- 1 packet stevia
- 1/2 tsp. cinnamon
- 2 oz. cream cheese
- 1 tbsp. coconut flour
- 1/2 tsp. vanilla

**Directions:**

1. Add all ingredients into the bowl and blend until smooth.
2. Spray pan with cooking spray and heat over medium-high heat.
3. Pour batter on the hot pan and make two pancakes.
4. Cook pancake until lightly brown from both the sides.
5. Serve and enjoy.

**Nutrition:**

Calories 386

Fat 30g

Carbohydrates 12g

Sugar 1g

Protein 16g

Cholesterol 389 mg

## 8. Cheesy Scrambled Eggs with Fresh Herbs

**Preparation Time:** 15 minutes

**Cooking Time:** 10 minutes

**Servings:** 4

**Ingredients:**

- Eggs – 3
- Egg whites – 2
- Cream cheese – 1/2 cup
- Unsweetened rice milk – 1/4 cup
- Chopped scallion – 1 Tbsp. green part only
- Chopped fresh tarragon – 1 Tbsp.
- Unsalted butter – 2 Tbsps.
- Ground black pepper to taste

**Directions:**

1. In a bowl, whisk the eggs, egg whites, cream cheese, rice milk, scallions, and tarragon until mixed and smooth.
2. Melt the butter in a skillet.
3. Pour in the egg mixture and cook, stirring, for 5 minutes or until the eggs are thick and curds creamy.
4. Season with pepper and serve.

**Nutrition:**

Calories: 221

Fat: 19g

Carb: 3g

Phosphorus: 119mg

Potassium: 140mg

Sodium: 193mg

Protein: 8g

## 9. Coconut Breakfast Smoothie

**Preparation Time:** 5 minutes

**Cooking Time:** 5 minutes

**Servings:** 1

**Ingredients:**

- 1/4 cup whey protein powder
- 1/2 cup coconut milk
- 5 drops liquid stevia
- 1 tbsp. coconut oil
- 1 tsp. vanilla
- 2 tbsp. coconut butter
- 1/4 cup water
- 1/2 cup ice

**Directions:**

1. Add all ingredients into the blender and blend until smooth.
2. Serve and enjoy.

**Nutrition:**

Calories 560

Fat 45g

Carbohydrates 12g

Sugar 4g

Protein 25g

Cholesterol 60 mg

## 10. Turkey and Green lettuce Scramble on Melba Toast

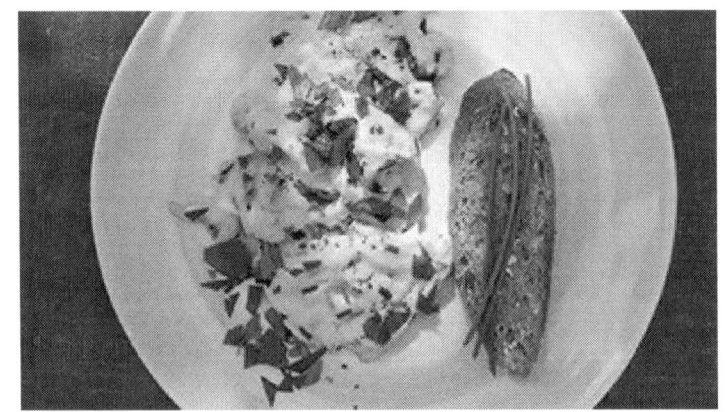

**Preparation Time:** 2 minutes
**Cooking Time:** 15 minutes
**Servings:** 2
**Ingredients:**

- Extra virgin olive oil – 1 tsp.
- Raw green lettuce – 1 cup
- Garlic – 1/2 clove, minced
- Nutmeg – 1 tsp. grated
- Cooked and diced turkey breast – 1 cup
- Melba toast – 4 slices
- Balsamic vinegar – 1 tsp.

**Directions:**

1. Heat a skillet over medium heat and add oil.
2. Add turkey and heat through for 6 to 8 minutes.
3. Add green lettuce, garlic, and nutmeg and stir-fry for 6 minutes more.
4. Plate up the Melba toast and top with green lettuce and turkey scramble.
5. Drizzle with balsamic vinegar and serve.

**Nutrition:**

Calories: 301
Fat: 19g
Carb: 12g
Phosphorus: 215mg
Potassium: 269mg
Sodium: 360mg
Protein: 19g

## 11. Vegetable Omelet

**Preparation Time:** 15 minutes
**Cooking Time:** 10 minutes
**Servings:** 3
**Ingredients:**

- Egg whites – 4
- Egg – 1
- Chopped fresh parsley – 2 Tbsps.
- Water – 2 Tbsps.
- Olive oil spray
- Chopped and boiled red bell pepper 1/2 cup
- Chopped scallion – 1/4 cup, both green and white parts
- Ground black pepper

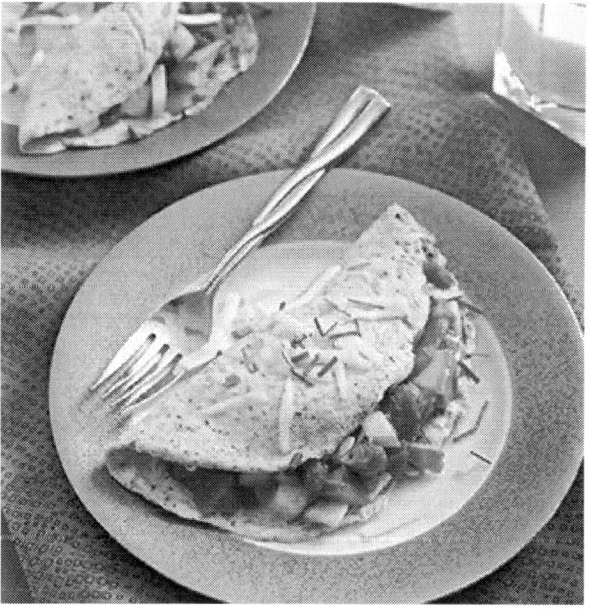

**Directions:**

1. Whisk together the egg, egg whites, parsley, and water until well blended. Set aside.
2. Spray a skillet with olive oil spray and place over medium heat.
3. Sauté the peppers and scallion for 3 minutes or until softened.
4. Pour the egg mixture into the skillet over vegetables and cook, swirling the skillet, for 2 minutes or until the edges start to set. Cook until set.
5. Season with black pepper and serve.

**Nutrition:**

Calories: 77
Fat: 3g
Carb: 2g
Phosphorus: 67mg
Potassium: 194mg
Sodium: 229mg
Protein: 12g

## 12. Mexican Style Burritos

**Preparation Time:** 5 minutes
**Cooking Time:** 15 minutes
**Servings:** 2
**Ingredients:**

- Olive oil – 1 Tbsp.
- Corn tortillas – 2
- Red onion – 1/4 cup, chopped
- Red bell peppers – 1/4 cup, chopped
- Red chili – 1/2, deseeded and chopped
- Eggs – 2
- Juice of 1 lime
- Cilantro – 1 Tbsp. chopped

**Directions:**

1. Turn the broiler to medium heat and place the tortillas underneath for 1 to 2 minutes on each side or until lightly toasted.
2. Remove and keep the broiler on.
3. Heat the oil in a skillet and sauté onion, chili and bell peppers for 5 to 6 minutes or until soft.
4. Crack the eggs over the top of the onions and peppers and place skillet under the broiler for 5 to 6 minutes or until the eggs are cooked.
5. Serve half the eggs and vegetables on top of each tortilla and sprinkle with cilantro and lime juice to serve.

**Nutrition:**
Calories: 202
Fat: 13g
Carb: 19g
Phosphorus: 184mg
Potassium: 233mg
Sodium: 77mg
Protein: 9g

## 13. Bulgur, Couscous and Buckwheat Cereal

**Preparation Time:** 10 minutes

**Cooking Time:** 25 minutes

**Servings:** 4

**Ingredients:**

- Water – 2 1/4 cups
- Vanilla rice milk – 1 1/4 cups
- Uncooked bulgur – 6 Tbsps.
- Uncooked whole buckwheat – 2 Tbsps.
- Sliced apple – 1 cup
- Plain uncooked couscous – 6 Tbsps.
- Ground cinnamon – 1/2 tsp.

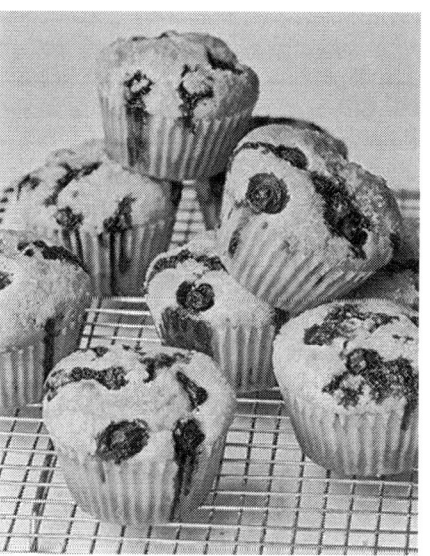

**Directions:**

1. In a saucepan, heat the water and milk over medium heat.
2. Bring to a boil, and add the bulgur, buckwheat, and apple.
3. Reduce the heat to low and simmer, occasionally stirring until the bulgur is tender, about 20 to 25 minutes.
4. Remove the saucepan from the heat and stir in the couscous and cinnamon.
5. Let the saucepan stand, covered, for 10 minutes.
6. Fluff the cereal with a fork before serving.

**Nutrition:**

Calories: 159

Fat: 1g

Carb: 34g

Phosphorus: 130mg

Potassium: 116mg

Sodium: 33mg

Protein: 4g

## 14. Sweet Pancakes

**Preparation Time:** 10 minutes

**Cooking Time:** 5 minutes

**Servings:** 5

**Ingredients:**

- All-purpose flour – 1 cup
- Granulated sugar – 1 Tbsp.
- Baking powder – 2 tsps.
- Egg whites – 2
- Almond milk - 1 cup
- Olive oil - 2 Tbsps.
- Maple extract – 1 Tbsp.

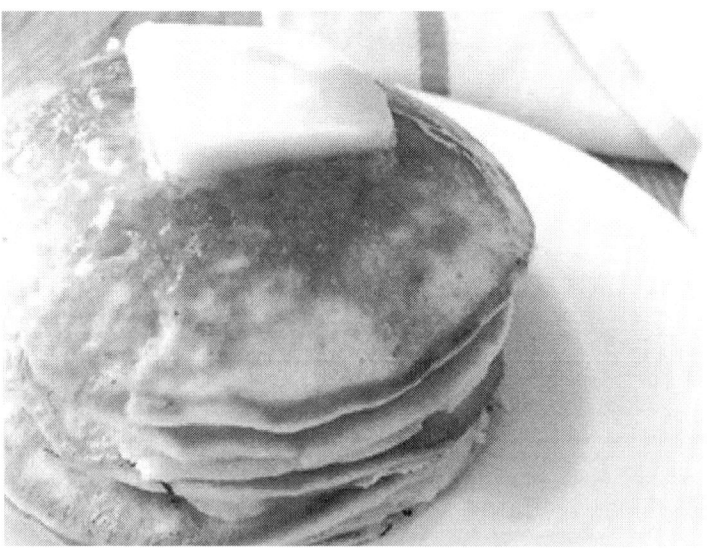

**Directions:**

1. Mix the flour, sugar and baking powder in a bowl.
2. Make a well in the center and place to one side.
3. In another bowl, mix the egg whites, milk, oil, and maple extract.
4. Add the egg mixture to the well and gently mix until a batter is formed.
5. Heat skillet over medium heat.
6. Add 1/5 of the batter to the pan and cook 2 minutes on each side or until the pancake is golden.
7. Repeat with the remaining batter and serve.

**Nutrition:**

Calories: 178

Fat: 6g

Carb: 25g

Phosphorus: 116mg

Potassium: 126mg

Sodium: 297mg

Protein: 6g

## 15. Breakfast Smoothie

**Preparation Time:** 15 minutes

**Cooking Time:** 0 minutes

**Servings:** 2

**Ingredients:**

- Frozen blueberries – 1 cup
- Pineapple chunks – 1/2 cup
- English cucumber – 1/2 cup
- Apple – 1/2
- Water – 1/2 cup

**Directions:**

1. Put the pineapple, blueberries, cucumber, apple, and water in a blender and blend until thick and smooth.
2. Pour into 2 glasses and serve.

**Nutrition:**

Calories: 87

Fat: g

Carb: 22g

Phosphorus: 28mg

Potassium: 192mg

Sodium: 3mg

Protein: 0.7g

## 16. Buckwheat and Grapefruit Porridge

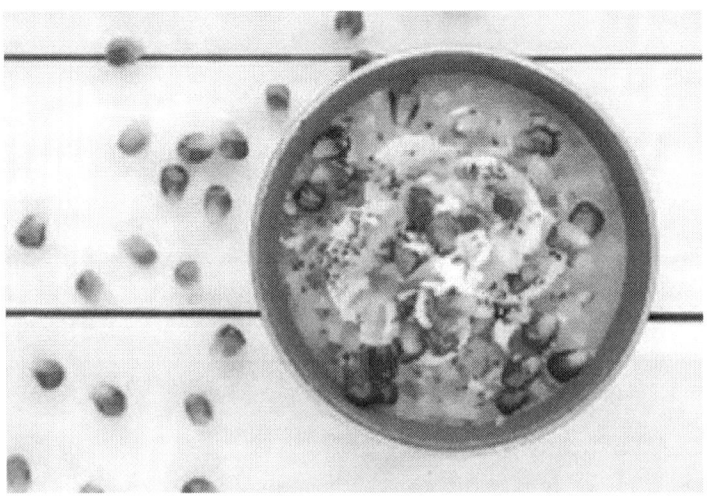

**Preparation Time:** 5 minutes

**Cooking Time:** 20 minutes

**Servings:** 2

**Ingredients:**

- Buckwheat – 1/2 cup
- Grapefruit – 1/4, chopped
- Honey – 1 Tbsp.
- Almond milk – 1 1/2 cups
- Water – 2 cups

**Directions:**

1. Bring the water to a boil on the stove. Add the buckwheat and place the lid on the pan.
2. Lower heat slightly and simmer for 7 to 10 minutes, checking to ensure water does not dry out.
3. When most of the water is absorbed, remove and set aside for 5 minutes.
4. Drain any excess water from the pan and stir in almond milk, heating through for 5 minutes.
5. Add the honey and grapefruit.
6. Serve.

**Nutrition:**

Calories: 231

Fat: 4g

Carb: 43g

Phosphorus: 165mg

Potassium: 370mg

Sodium: 135mg

## 17. Egg and Veggie Muffins

**Preparation Time:** 15 minutes
**Cooking Time:** 20 minutes
**Servings:** 4
**Ingredients:**

- Cooking spray
- Eggs – 4
- Unsweetened rice milk – 2 Tbsp.
- Sweet onion – 1/2, chopped
- Red bell pepper – 1/2, chopped
- Pinch red pepper flakes
- Pinch ground black pepper

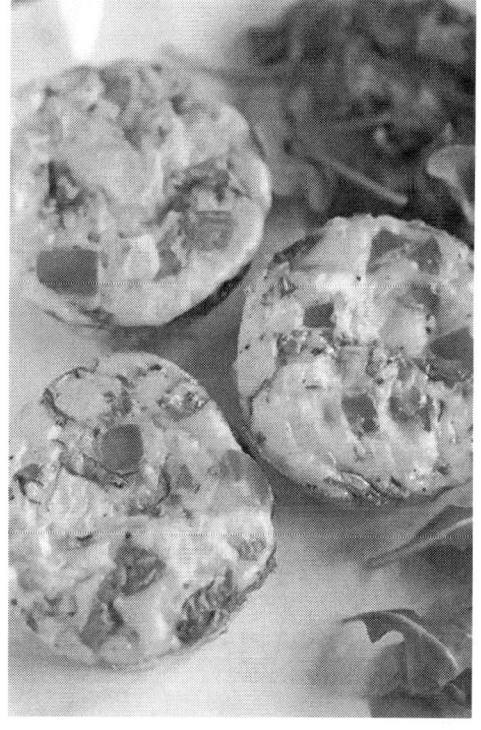

**Directions:**

1. Preheat the oven to 350F.
2. Spray 4 muffin pans with cooking spray. Set aside.
3. In a bowl, whisk together the milk, eggs, onion, red pepper, parsley, red pepper flakes, and black pepper until mixed.
4. Pour the egg mixture into prepared muffin pans.
5. Bake until the muffins are puffed and golden, about 18 to 20 minutes.
6. serve

**Nutrition:**

Calories: 84

Fat: 5g

Carb: 3g

Phosphorus: 110mg

Potassium: 117mg

Sodium: 75mg

Protein: 7g

## 18. Salad with Vinaigrette

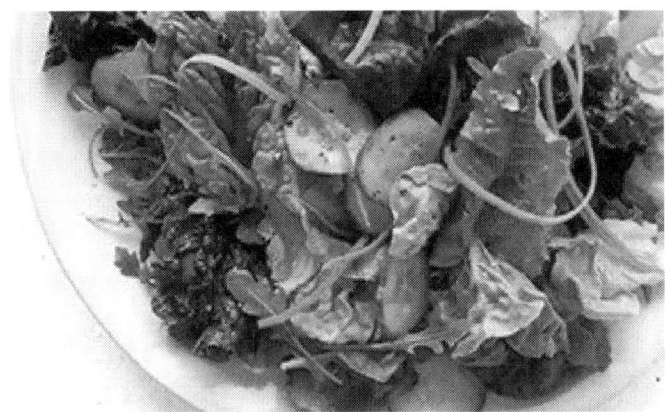

**Preparation Time:** 25 minutes

**Cooking Time:** 0 minutes

**Servings:** 4

**Ingredients:**

For the vinaigrette:

- Olive oil – 1/2 cup
- Balsamic vinegar - 4 Tbsps.
- Chopped fresh oregano – 2 Tbsps.
- Pinch red pepper flakes
- Ground black pepper

For the salad

- Shredded green leaf lettuce – 4 cups
- Carrot – 1, shredded
- Fresh green beans – ¾ cup, cut into 1-inch pieces
- Large radishes – 3, sliced thin

**Directions:**

1. To make the vinaigrette: put the vinaigrette Ingredients in a bowl and whisk.
2. To make the salad, in a bowl, toss together the carrot, lettuce, green beans, and radishes.
3. Add the vinaigrette to the vegetables and toss to coat.
4. Arrange the salad on plates and serve.

**Nutrition:**

Calories: 273

Fat: 27g

Carb: 7g

Phosphorus: 30mg

Potassium: 197mg

Sodium: 27mg

Protein: 1g

## 19. Salad with Lemon Dressing

**Preparation Time:** 10 minutes

**Cooking Time:** 0 minutes

**Servings:** 4

**Ingredients:**

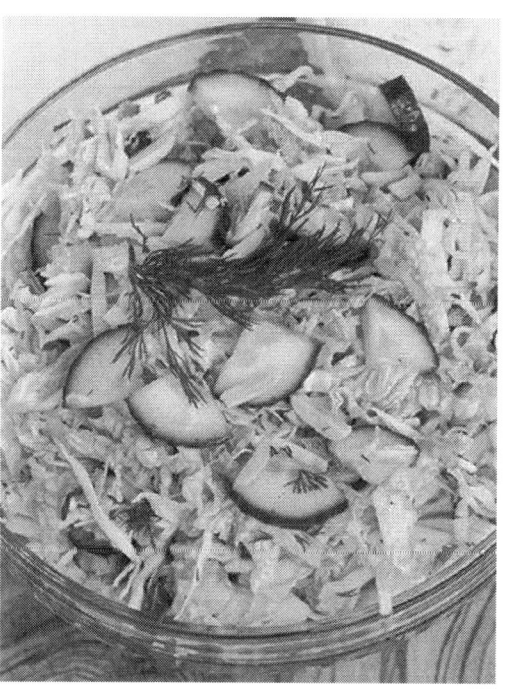

- Heavy cream – 1/4 cup
- Freshly squeezed lemon juice – 1/4 cup
- Granulated sugar – 2 Tbsps.
- Chopped fresh dill – 2 Tbsps.
- Finely chopped scallion – 2 Tbsps. green part only
- Ground black pepper – 1/4 tsp.
- English cucumber – 1, sliced thin
- Shredded green cabbage – 2 cups

**Directions:**

1. In a small bowl, stir together the lemon juice, cream, sugar, dill, scallion, and pepper until well blended.
2. In a large bowl, toss together the cucumber and cabbage.
3. Place the salad in the refrigerator and chill for 1 hour.
4. Stir before serving.

**Nutrition:**

Calories: 99

Fat: 6g

Carb: 13g

Phosphorus: 38mg

Potassium: 200mg

Sodium: 14mg

Protein: 2g

## 20. Shrimp with Salsa

**Preparation Time:** 15 minutes

**Cooking Time:** 10 minutes

**Servings:** 4

**Ingredients:**

- Olive oil – 2 Tbsp.
- Large shrimp – 6 ounces, peeled and deveined, tails left on
- Minced garlic – 1 tsp.
- Chopped English cucumber – 1/2 cup
- Chopped mango – 1/2 cup
- Zest of 1 lime
- Juice of 1 lime
- Ground black pepper
- Lime wedges for garnish

**Directions:**

1. Soak 4 wooden skewers in water for 30 minutes.
2. Preheat the barbecue to medium heat.
3. In a bowl, toss together the olive oil, shrimp, and garlic.
4. Thread the shrimp onto the skewers, about 4 shrimp per skewer.
5. In a bowl, stir together the mango, cucumber, lime zest, and lime juice, and season the salsa lightly with pepper. Set aside.
6. Grill the shrimp for 10 minutes, turning once or until the shrimp is opaque and cooked through.
7. Season the shrimp lightly with pepper.
8. Serve the shrimp on the cucumber salsa with lime wedges on the side.

**Nutrition:**

Calories: 120

Fat: 8g

Carb: 4g

Phosphorus: 91mg

Potassium: 129mg

Sodium: 60mg

Protein: 9g

## 21. Pesto Pork Chops

**Preparation Time:** 20 minutes
**Cooking Time:** 20 minutes
**Servings:** 4
**Ingredients:**

- Pork top-loin chops – 4 (3-ounce) boneless, fat trimmed
- Herb pesto – 8 tsps.
- Breadcrumbs – 1/2 cup
- Olive oil – 1 Tbsp.

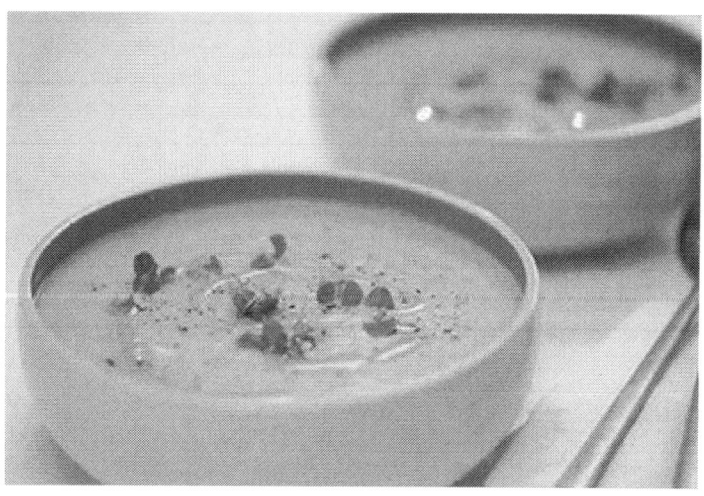

**Directions:**

1. Preheat the oven to 450F.
2. Line a baking sheet with foil. Set aside.
3. Rub 1 tsp. of pesto evenly over both sides of each pork chop.
4. Lightly dredge each pork chop in the breadcrumbs.
5. Heat the oil in a skillet.
6. Brown the pork chops on each side for 5 minutes.
7. Place the pork chops on the baking sheet.
8. Bake for 10 minutes or until pork reaches 145F in the center.

**Nutrition:**

Calories: 210
Fat: 7g
Carb: 10g
Phosphorus: 179mg
Potassium: 220mg
Sodium: 148mg
Protein: 24g

## 22. Turkey Burgers

**Preparation Time:** 15 minutes

**Cooking Time:** 8 minutes

**Servings:** 5

**Ingredients:**

- 1 ripe pear, peeled, cored and chopped roughly
- 1-pound lean ground turkey
- 1 teaspoon fresh ginger, grated finely
- 2 minced garlic cloves
- 1 teaspoon fresh rosemary, minced
- 1 teaspoon fresh sage, minced
- Salt, to taste
- Freshly ground black pepper, to taste
- 1-2 tablespoons coconut oil

**Directions:**

1. In a blender, add pear and pulse till smooth.
2. Transfer the pear mixture in a large bowl with remaining ingredients except for oil and mix till well combined.
3. Make small equal sized 10 patties from the mixture.
4. In a heavy-bottomed frying pan, heat oil on medium heat.
5. Add the patties and cook for around 4-5 minutes.
6. Flip the inside and cook for approximately 2-3 minutes.

**Nutrition:**

Calories: 477

Fat: 15g

Carbohydrates: 26g

Fiber: 11g

Protein: 35g

# CHAPTER 6:

# Lunch

## 23. Dolmas Wrap

**Preparation Time:** 10 minutes

**Cooking Time:** 5 minutes

**Servings:** 2

**Ingredients:**
- 2 whole wheat wraps
- 6 dolmas (stuffed grape leaves)
- 1 tomato, chopped
- 1 cucumber, chopped
- 2 oz. Greek yogurt
- ½ teaspoon minced garlic
- ¼ cup lettuce, chopped
- 2 oz. Feta, crumbled

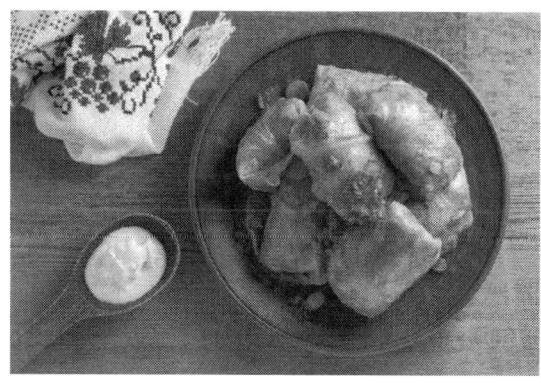

**Directions:**

1. In the mixing bowl combine together chopped tomato, cucumber, Greek yogurt, minced garlic, lettuce, and Feta.
2. When the mixture is homogenous transfer it in the center of every wheat wrap.
3. Arrange dolma over the vegetable mixture.
4. Carefully wrap the wheat wraps.

**Nutrition:** calories 341, fat 12.9, fiber 9.2, carbs 52.4, protein 13.2 Phosphorus: 110mg Potassium: 117mg Sodium: 75mg

## 24. Salad al Tonno

**Preparation Time: 15 minutes**

**Cooking Time: 0 minutes**

**Servings: 2**

**Ingredients:**

- 1 ½ cup lettuce leaves, teared
- ½ cup cherry Red bell peppers, halved
- ½ teaspoon garlic powder
- ½ teaspoon salt
- ½ teaspoon ground black pepper
- 1 tablespoon lemon juice
- 6 oz. tuna, canned, drained

**Directions:**

1. Chop the tuna roughly and put it in the salad bowl.
2. Add cherry Red bell peppers, lettuce leaves, salt, garlic powder, ground black pepper. Lemon juice, and olive oil.
4. Give a good shake to the salad.
5. Salad can be stored in the fridge for up to 3 hours.

**Nutrition:** calories 235, fat 12, fiber 1, carbs 6.5, protein 23.4 Phosphorus: 120mg Potassium: 217mg Sodium: 75mg

## 25. Arlecchino Rice Salad

**Preparation Time: 10 minutes**

**Cooking Time: 15 minutes**

**Servings: 3**

**Ingredients:**

- ½ cup white rice, dried
- 1 cup chicken stock
- 1 zucchini, shredded
- 2 tablespoons capers
- 1 carrot, shredded
- 1 tomato, chopped
- 1 tablespoon apple cider vinegar
- ½ teaspoon salt
- 2 tablespoons fresh parsley, chopped
- 1 tablespoon canola oil

**Directions:**

1. Put rice in the pan.
2. Add chicken stock and boil it with the closed lid for 15-20 minutes or until rice absorbs all water.
3. Meanwhile, in the mixing bowl combine together shredded zucchini, capers, carrot, and tomato.
4. Add fresh parsley.
5. Make the dressing: mix up together canola oil, salt, and apple cider vinegar.
6. Chill the cooked rice little and add it in the salad bowl to the vegetables.
7. Add dressing and mix up salad well.

**Nutrition:** calories 183, fat 5.3, fiber 2.1, carbs 30.4, protein 3.8 Phosphorus: 110mg Potassium: 117mg Sodium: 75mg

## 26. Sauteed Chickpea and Lentil Mix

**Preparation Time: 10 minutes**

**Cooking Time: 50 minutes**

**Servings: 4**

**Ingredients:**

- 1 cup chickpeas, half-cooked
- 1 cup lentils
- 5 cups chicken stock
- ½ cup fresh cilantro, chopped
- 1 teaspoon salt
- ½ teaspoon chili flakes
- ¼ cup onion, diced
- 1 tablespoon tomato paste

**Directions:**

1. Place chickpeas in the pan.
2. Add water, salt, and chili flakes.
3. Boil the chickpeas for 30 minutes over the medium heat.
4. Then add diced onion, lentils, and tomato paste. Stir well.
5. Close the lid and cook the mix for 15 minutes.
6. After this, add chopped cilantro, stir the meal well and cook it for 5 minutes more.
7. Let the cooked lunch chill little before serving.

**Nutrition:** calories 370, fat 4.3, fiber 23.7, carbs 61.6, protein 23.2 Phosphorus: 110mg Potassium: 117mg Sodium: 75mg

## 27. Crazy Japanese Potato and Beef Croquettes

**Preparation Time: 10 minutes**

**Cooking Time: 20 minutes**

**Servings: 10**

**Ingredients:**

- 3 medium russet potatoes, peeled and chopped
- 1 tablespoon almond butter
- 1 tablespoon vegetable oil
- 3 onions, diced
- ¾ pound ground beef
- 4 teaspoons light coconut aminos
- All-purpose flour for coating
- 2 eggs, beaten
- Panko bread crumbs for coating
- ½ cup oil, frying

**Directions:**

1. Take a saucepan and place it over medium-high heat; add potatoes and sunflower seeds water, boil for 16 minutes.
2. Remove water and put potatoes in another bowl, add almond butter and mash the potatoes.
3. Take a frying pan and place it over medium heat, add 1 tablespoon oil and let it heat up.
4. Add onions and stir fry until tender.
5. Add coconut aminos to beef to onions.
6. Keep frying until beef is browned.
7. Mix the beef with the potatoes evenly.
8. Take another frying pan and place it over medium heat; add half a cup of oil.
9. Form croquettes using the mashed potato mixture and coat them with flour, then eggs and finally breadcrumbs.
10. Fry patties until golden on all sides.
11. Enjoy!

**Nutrition:** Calories: 239 Fat: 4g Carbohydrates: 20g Protein: 10g Phosphorus: 120mg Potassium: 107mg Sodium: 75mg

## 28. Traditional Black Bean Chili

**Preparation Time: 10 minutes**

**Cooking Time: 4 hours**

**Servings: 4**

**Ingredients:**

- 1 ½ cups red bell pepper, chopped
- 1 cup yellow onion, chopped
- 1 ½ cups mushrooms, sliced
- 1 tablespoon olive oil
- 1 tablespoon chili powder
- 2 garlic cloves, minced
- 1 teaspoon chipotle chili pepper, chopped
- ½ teaspoon cumin, ground
- 16 ounces canned black beans, drained and rinsed
- 2 tablespoons cilantro, chopped
- 1 cup Red bell peppers, chopped

**Directions:**

1. Add red bell peppers, onion, dill, mushrooms, chili powder, garlic, chili pepper, cumin, black beans, and Red bell peppers to your Slow Cooker.
2. Stir well.
3. Place lid and cook on HIGH for 4 hours.
4. Sprinkle cilantro on top.
5. Serve and enjoy!

**Nutrition:** Calories: 211 Fat: 3g Carbohydrates: 22g Protein: 5g Phosphorus: 90mg Potassium: 107mg Sodium: 75mg

## 29. Green Palak Paneer

**Preparation Time:** 5 minutes

**Cooking Time:** 10 minutes

**Servings:** 4

**Ingredients:**

- 1-pound green lettuce
- 2 cups cubed paneer (vegan)
- 2 tablespoons coconut oil
- 1 teaspoon cumin
- 1 chopped up onion
- 1-2 teaspoons hot green chili minced up
- 1 teaspoon minced garlic
- 15 cashews
- 4 tablespoons almond milk
- 1 teaspoon Garam masala
- Flavored vinegar as needed

**Directions:**

1. Add cashews and milk to a blender and blend well.
2. Set your pot to Sauté mode and add coconut oil; allow the oil to heat up.
3. Add cumin seeds, garlic, green chilies, ginger and sauté for 1 minute.
4. Add onion and sauté for 2 minutes.
5. Add chopped green lettuce, flavored vinegar and a cup of water.
6. Lock up the lid and cook on HIGH pressure for 10 minutes.
7. Quick-release the pressure.
8. Add ½ cup of water and blend to a paste.
9. Add cashew paste, paneer and Garam Masala and stir thoroughly.
10. Serve over hot rice!

**Nutrition:** Calories: 367 Fat: 26g Carbohydrates: 21g Protein: 16g Phosphorus: 110mg Potassium: 117mg Sodium: 75mg

## 30. Cucumber Sandwich

**Preparation Time: 1 hour**
**Cooking Time: 5 minutes**
**Servings: 2**
**Ingredients:**

- 6 tsp. of cream cheese
- 1 pinch of dried dill weed
- 3 tsp. of mayonnaise
- .25 tsp. dry Italian dressing mix
- 4 slices of white bread
- .5 of a cucumber

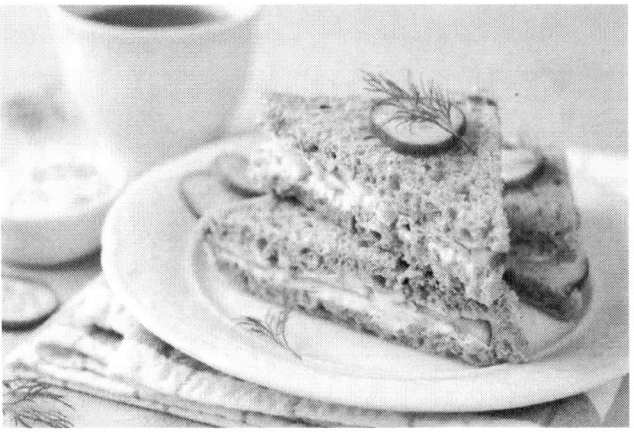

**Directions:**

1. Prepare the cucumber and cut it into slices.
2. Mix cream cheese, mayonnaise, and Italian dressing. Chill for one hour.
3. Distribute the mixture onto the white bread slices.
4. Place cucumber slices on top and sprinkle with the dill weed.
5. Cut in halves and serve.

**Nutrition:**

Calories: 143

Fat: 6g

Carbs: 16.7g

Protein: 4g

Sodium: 255mg

Potassium: 127mg

Phosphorus: 64mg

## 31. Pizza Pitas

**Preparation Time: 10 minutes**
**Cooking Time: 10 minutes**
**Servings: 1**
**Ingredients:**

- .33 cup of mozzarella cheese
- 2 pieces of pita bread, 6 inches in size
- 6 tsp. of chunky tomato sauce
- 2 cloves of garlic (minced)
- .25 cups of onion, chopped small
- .25 tsp. of red pepper flakes
- .25 cup of bell pepper, chopped small
- 2 ounces of ground pork, lean
- No-stick oil spray
- .5 tsp. of fennel seeds

**Directions:**

1. Preheat oven to 400.
2. Put the garlic, ground meat, pepper flakes, onion, and bell pepper in a pan. Sauté until cooked.
3. Grease a flat baking pan and put pitas on it. Use the mixture to spread on the pita bread.
4. Spread one tablespoon of the tomato sauce and top with cheese.
5. Bake for five to eight minutes, until the cheese is bubbling.

**Nutrition:**

Calories: 284

Fat: 10g

Carbs: 34g

Protein: 16g

Sodium: 795mg

Potassium: 706mg

Phosphorus: 416mg

## 32. Lettuce Wraps with Chicken

**Preparation Time: 10 minutes**
**Cooking Time: 15 minutes**
**Servings: 4**
**Ingredients:**

- 8 lettuce leaves
- .25 cups of fresh cilantro
- .25 cups of mushroom
- 1 tsp. of five spices seasoning
- .25 cups of onion
- 6 tsp. of rice vinegar
- 2 tsp. of hoisin
- 6 tsp. of oil (canola)
- 3 tsp. of oil (sesame)
- 2 tsp. of garlic
- 2 scallions
- 8 ounces of cooked chicken breast

**Directions:**

1. Mince together the cooked chicken and the garlic. Chop up the onions, cilantro, mushrooms, and scallions.
2. Use a skillet overheat, combine chicken to all remaining ingredients, minus the lettuce leaves. Cook for fifteen minutes, stirring occasionally.
3. Place .25 cups of the mixture into each leaf of lettuce.
4. Wrap the lettuce around like a burrito and eat.

**Nutrition:**

Calories: 84

Fat: 4g

Carbs: 9g

Protein: 5.9g

Sodium: 618mg

Potassium: 258mg

Phosphorus: 64mg

## 33. Turkey Pinwheels

**Preparation Time:** 10 minutes

**Cooking Time:** 15 minutes

**Servings:** 6

**Ingredients:**

- 6 toothpicks
- 8 oz. of spring mix salad greens
- 1 ten-inch tortilla
- 2 ounces of thinly sliced deli turkey
- 9 tsp. of whipped cream cheese
- 1 roasted red bell pepper

**Directions:**

1. Cut the red bell pepper into ten strips about a quarter-inch thick.
2. Spread the whipped cream cheese on the tortilla evenly.
3. Add the salad greens to create a base layer and then lay the turkey on top of it.
4. Space out the red bell pepper strips on top of the turkey.
5. Tuck the end and begin rolling the tortilla inward.
6. Use the toothpicks to hold the roll into place and cut it into six pieces.
7. Serve with the swirl facing upward.

**Nutrition:**

Calories: 206

Fat: 9g

Carbs: 21g

Protein: 9g

Sodium: 533mg

Potassium: 145mg

Phosphorus: 47mg

## 34. Chicken Tacos

**Preparation Time:** 5 minutes

**Cooking Time:** 20 minutes

**Servings:** 4

**Ingredients:**
- 8 corn tortillas
- 1.5 tsp. of Sodium-free taco seasoning
- 1 juiced lime
- .5 cups of cilantro
- 2 green onions, chopped
- 8 oz. of iceberg or romaine lettuce, shredded or chopped
- .25 cup of sour cream
- 1 pound of boneless and skinless chicken breast

**Directions:**
1. Cook chicken, by boiling, for twenty minutes. Shred or chop cooked chicken into fine bite-sized pieces.
2. Mix the seasoning and lime juice with the chicken.
3. Put chicken mixture and lettuce in tortillas.
4. Top with the green onions, cilantro, and sour cream.

**Nutrition:**

Calories: 260

Fat: 3g

Carbs: 36g

Protein: 23g

Sodium: 922mg

Potassium: 445mg

Phosphorus: 357mg

## 35. Tuna Twist

**Preparation Time:** 10 minutes
**Cooking Time:** 30 minutes
**Servings:** 4

**Ingredients:**

- 1 can of unsalted or water packaged tuna, drained
- 6 tsp. of vinegar
- .5 cup of cooked peas
- .5 cup celery (chopped)
- 3 tsp. of dried dill weed
- 12 oz. cooked macaroni
- .75 cup of mayonnaise

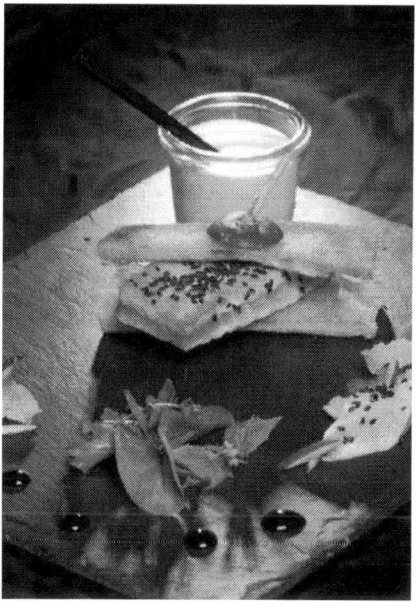

**Directions:**

1. Stir together the macaroni, vinegar, and mayonnaise together until blended and smooth.
2. Stir in remaining ingredients.
3. Chill before serving.

**Nutrition:**

Calories: 290

Fat: 10g

Carbs: 32g

Protein: 16g

Sodium: 307mg

Potassium: 175mg

Phosphorus: 111mg

## 36. Ciabatta Rolls with Chicken Pesto

**Preparation Time: 10 minutes**

**Cooking Time: 20 minutes**

**Servings: 2**

**Ingredients:**

- 6 tsp. of Greek yogurt
- 6 tsp. of pesto
- 2 small ciabatta rolls
- 8 oz. of a shredded iceberg or romaine lettuce
- 8 oz. of cooked boneless and skinless chicken breast, shredded
- .125 tsp. of pepper

**Directions:**

1. Combine the shredded chicken, pesto, pepper, and Greek yogurt in a medium-sized bowl.
2. Slice and toast the ciabatta rolls.
3. Divide the shredded chicken and pesto mixture in half and make sandwiches with the ciabatta rolls.
4. Top with shredded lettuce if desired.

**Nutrition:**

Calories: 374

Fat: 10g

Carbs: 40g

Protein: 30g

Sodium: 522mg

Potassium: 360mg

Phosphorus: 84mg

## 37. Marinated Shrimp Pasta Salad

**Preparation Time:** 15 minutes

**Cooking Time:** 5 hours

**Servings:** 1

**Ingredients:**

- 1/4 cup of honey
- 1/4 cup of balsamic vinegar
- 1/2 of an English cucumber, cubed
- 1/2 pound of fully cooked shrimp
- 15 baby carrots
- 1.5 cups of dime-sized cut cauliflower
- 4 stalks of celery, diced
- 1/2 large yellow bell pepper (diced)
- 1/2 red onion (diced)
- 1/2 large red bell pepper (diced)
- 12 ounces of uncooked tri-color pasta (cooked)
- 3/4 cup of olive oil
- 3 tsp. of mustard (Dijon)
- 1/2 tsp. of garlic (powder)
- 1/2 tsp. pepper

**Directions:**

1. Cut vegetables and put them in a bowl with the shrimp.
2. Whisk together the honey, balsamic vinegar, garlic powder, pepper, and Dijon mustard in a small bowl. While still whisking, slowly add the oil and whisk it all together.
3. Add the cooked pasta to the bowl with the shrimp and vegetables and mix it.
4. Toss the sauce to coat the pasta, shrimp, and vegetables evenly.
5. Cover and chill for a minimum of five hours before serving. Stir and serve while chilled.

**Nutrition:**

Calories: 205

Fat: 13g

Carbs: 10g

Protein: 12g

Sodium: 363mg

Potassium: 156mg

Phosphorus: 109mg

## 38. Peanut Butter and Jelly Grilled Sandwich

**Preparation Time: 5 minutes**

**Cooking Time: 5 minutes**

**Servings: 1**

**Ingredients:**

- 2 tsp. butter (unsalted)
- 6 tsp. butter (peanut)
- 3 tsp. of flavored jelly
- 2 pieces of bread

**Directions:**

1. Put the peanut butter evenly on one bread. Add the layer of jelly.
2. Butter the outside of the pieces of bread.
3. Add the sandwich to a frying pan and toast both sides.

**Nutrition:**

Calories: 300

Fat: 7g

Carbs: 49g

Protein: 8g

Sodium: 460mg

Potassium: 222mg

Phosphorus: 80mg

## 39. Grilled Onion and Pepper Jack Grilled Cheese Sandwich

**Preparation Time:** 5 minutes

**Cooking Time:** 5 minutes

**Servings:** 2

**Ingredients:**

- 1 tsp. of oil (olive)
- 6 tsp. of whipped cream cheese
- 1/2 of a medium onion
- 2 ounces of pepper jack cheese
- 4 slices of rye bread
- 2 tsp. of unsalted butter

**Directions:**

1. Set out the butter so that it becomes soft. Slice up the onion into thin slices.
2. Sauté onion slices. Continue to stir until cooked. Remove and put it to the side.
3. Spread one tablespoon of the whipped cream cheese on two of the slices of bread.
4. Then add grilled onions and cheese to each slice. Then top using the other two bread slices.
5. Spread the softened butter on the outside of the slices of bread.
6. Use the skillet to toast the sandwiches until lightly brown and the cheese is melted.

**Nutrition:**

Calories: 350

Fat: 18g

Carbs: 34g

Protein: 13g

Sodium: 589mg

Potassium: 184mg

Phosphorus: 226mg

## 40. Crispy Lemon Chicken

**Preparation Time:** 10 minutes

**Cooking Time:** 10 minutes

**Servings:** 6

**Ingredients:**

- 1 lb. boneless and skinless chicken breast
- ½ cup of all-purpose flour
- 1 large egg
- ½ cup of lemon juice
- 2 tbsp. of water
- ¼ tsp salt
- ¼ tsp lemon pepper
- 1 tsp of mixed herb seasoning
- 2 tbsp. of olive oil
- A few lemon slices for garnishing
- 1 tbsp. of chopped parsley (for garnishing)
- 2 cups of cooked plain white rice

**Directions:**

1. Slice the chicken breast into thin and season with the herb, salt, and pepper.
2. In a small bowl, whisk together the egg with the water.
3. Keep the flour in a separate bowl.
4. Dip the chicken slices in the egg bath and then into the flour.
5. Heat your oil in a medium frying pan.
6. Shallow fry the chicken in the pan until golden brown.
7. Add the lemon juice and cook for another couple of minutes.
8. Taken the chicken out of the pan and transfer on a wide dish with absorbing paper to absorb any excess oil.
9. Garnish with some chopped parsley and lemon wedges on top.
10. Serve with rice.

**Nutrition:**

Calories: 232 Carbohydrate: 24g

Protein: 18g Fat: 8g

Sodium: 100g Potassium: 234mg Phosphorus: 217mg

## 41. Mexican Steak Tacos

**Preparation Time:** 10 minutes

**Cooking Time:** 15 minutes

**Servings:** 8

**Ingredients:**

- 1 pound of flank or skirt steak
- ¼ cup of fresh cilantro, chopped
- ¼ cup white onion, chopped
- 3 limes, juiced
- 3 cloves of garlic, minced
- 2 tsp of garlic powder
- 2 tbsp. of olive oil
- ½ cup of Mexican or mozzarella cheese, grated
- 1 tsp of Mexican seasoning
- 8 medium-sized (6") corn flour tortillas

**Directions:**

1. Combine the juice from two limes, Mexican seasoning, and garlic powder in a dish or bowl and marinate the steak with it for at least half an hour in the fridge.
2. In a separate bowl, combine the chopped cilantro, garlic, onion, and juice from one lime to make your salsa. Cover and keep in the fridge.
3. Slice steak into thin strips and cook for approximately 3 minutes on each side.
4. Preheat your oven to 350F/180C.
5. Distribute evenly the steak strips in each tortilla. Top with a tablespoon of the grated cheese on top.
6. Wrap each taco in aluminum foil and bake in the oven for 7-8 minutes or until cheese is melted.
7. Serve warm with your cilantro salsa.

**Nutrition:**

Calories: 230

Carbohydrate: 19.5 g

Protein: 15 g

Fat: 11 g

Sodium: 486.75 g

Potassium: 240 mg

Phosphorus: 268 mg

## 42. Beer Pork Ribs

**Preparation Time:** 10 minutes

**Cooking Time:** 8 hours

**Servings:** 1

**Ingredients:**

- 2 pounds of pork ribs, cut into two units/racks
- 18 oz. of root beer
- 2 cloves of garlic, minced
- 2 tbsp. of onion powder
- 2 tbsp. of vegetable oil (optional)

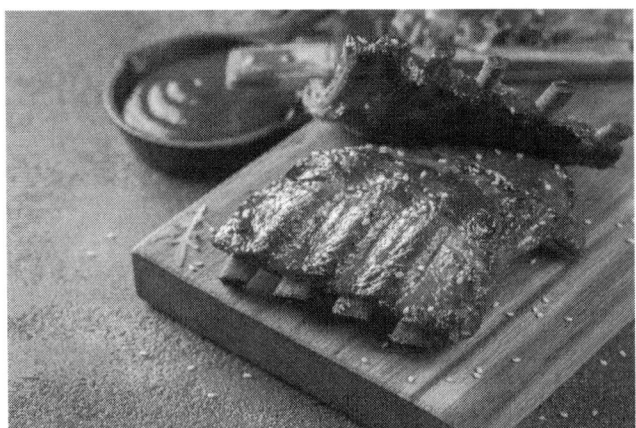

**Directions:**

1. Wrap the pork ribs with vegetable oil and place one unit on the bottom of your slow cooker with half of the minced garlic and the onion powder.
2. Place the other rack on top with the rest of the garlic and onion powder.
3. Pour over the root beer and cover the lid.
4. Let simmer for 8 hours on low heat.
5. Take off and finish optionally in a grilling pan for a nice sear.

**Nutrition:**

Calories: 301

Carbohydrate: 36 g

Protein: 21 g

Fat: 18 g

Sodium: 729 mg

Potassium: 200 mg

Phosphorus: 209 mg

## 43. Mexican Chorizo Sausage

**Preparation Time: 10 minutes**

**Cooking Time: 15 minutes**

**Servings: 1**

**Ingredients:**

- 2 pounds of boneless pork but coarsely ground
- 3 tbsp. of red wine vinegar
- 2 tbsp. of smoked paprika
- ½ tsp of cinnamon
- ½ tsp of ground cloves
- ¼ tsp of coriander seeds
- ¼ tsp ground ginger
- 1 tsp of ground cumin
- 3 tbsp. of brandy

**Directions:**

1. In a large mixing bowl, combine the ground pork with the seasonings, brandy, and vinegar and mix with your hands well.
2. Place the mixture into a large Ziploc bag and leave in the fridge overnight.
3. Form into 15-16 patties of equal size.
4. Heat the oil in a large pan and fry the patties for 5-7 minutes on each side, or until the meat inside is no longer pink and there is a light brown crust on top.
5. Serve hot.

**Nutrition:**

Calories: 134

Carbohydrate: 0 g

Protein: 10 g

Fat: 7 g

Sodium: 40 mg

Potassium: 138 mg

Phosphorus: 128 mg

## 44. Eggplant Casserole

**Preparation Time:** 10 minutes

**Cooking Time:** 25 – 30 minutes

**Servings:** 4

**Ingredients:**

- 3 cups of eggplant, peeled and cut into large chunks
- 2 egg whites
- 1 large egg, whole
- ½ cup of unsweetened vegetable
- ¼ tsp of sage
- ½ cup of breadcrumbs
- 1 tbsp. of margarine, melted
- 1/4 tsp garlic salt

**Directions:**

1. Preheat the oven at 350F/180C.
2. Place the eggplants chunks in a medium pan, cover with a bit of water and cook with the lid covered until tender. Drain from the water and mash with a tool or fork.
3. Beat the eggs with the non-dairy vegetable cream, sage, salt, and pepper. Whisk in the eggplant mush.
4. Combine the melted margarine with the breadcrumbs.
5. Bake in the oven for 20-25 minutes or until the casserole has a golden-brown crust.

**Nutrition:**

Calories: 186

Carbohydrate: 19 g

Protein: 7 g

Fat: 9 g

Sodium: 503 mg

Potassium: 230 mg

Phosphorus: 62 mg

## 45. Pizza with Chicken and Pesto

**Preparation Time:** 10 minutes

**Cooking Time:** 25 minutes

**Servings:** 4

**Ingredients:**

- 1 ready-made frozen pizza dough
- 2/3 cup cooked chicken, chopped
- 1/2 cup of orange bell pepper, diced
- 1/2 cup of green bell pepper, diced
- 1/4 cup of purple onion, chopped
- 2 tbsp. of green basil pesto
- 1 tbsp. of chives, chopped
- 1/3 cup of parmesan or Romano cheese, grated
- 1/4 cup of mozzarella cheese
- 1 tbsp. of olive oil

**Directions:**

1. Thaw the pizza dough according to instructions on the package.
2. Heat the olive oil in a pan and sauté the peppers and onions for a couple of minutes. Set aside
3. Once the pizza dough has thawed, spread the Bali pesto over its surface.
4. Top with half of the cheese, the peppers, the onions, and the chicken. Finish with the rest of the cheese.
5. Bake at 350F/180C for approx. 20 minutes (or until crust and cheese are baked).
6. Slice in triangles with a pizza cutter or sharp knife and serve.

**Nutrition:**

Calories: 225

Carbohydrate: 13.9 g

Protein: 11.1 g

Fat: 12 g

Sodium: 321 mg

Potassium: 174 mg

Phosphorus: 172 mg

## 46. Shrimp Quesadilla

**Preparation Time:** 10 minutes

**Cooking Time:** 10 minutes

Servings: 2

**Ingredients:**

- 5 oz. of shrimp, shelled and deveined
- 4 tbsp. of Mexican salsa
- 2 tbsp. of fresh cilantro, chopped
- 1 tbsp. of lemon juice
- 1 tsp of ground cumin
- 1 tsp of cayenne pepper
- 2 tbsp. of unsweetened soy yogurt or creamy tofu
- 2 medium corn flour tortillas
- 2 tbsp. of low-fat cheddar cheese

**Directions:**

1. Mix the cilantro, cumin, lemon juice, and cayenne in a Ziploc bag to make your marinade.
2. Put the shrimps and marinate for 10 minutes.
3. Heat a pan over medium heat with some olive oil and toss in the shrimp with the marinade. Let cook for a couple of minutes or as soon as shrimps have turned pink and opaque.
4. Add the soy cream or soft tofu to the pan and mix well. Remove from the heat and keep the marinade aside.
5. Heat tortillas in the grill or microwave for a few seconds.
6. Place 2 tbsp. of salsa on each tortilla. Top one tortilla with the shrimp mixture and add the cheese on top.
7. Stack one tortilla against each other (with the spread salsa layer facing the shrimp mixture).
8. Transfer this on a baking tray and cook for 7-8 minutes at 350F/180C to melt the cheese and crisp up the tortillas.
9. Serve warm.

**Nutrition:**

Calories: 255

Carbohydrate: 21 g

Fat: 9 g

Protein: 24 g Sodium: 562 g

Potassium: 235 mg

Phosphorus: 189 mg

## 47. Grilled Corn on the Cob

**Preparation Time: 5 minutes**

**Cooking Time: 20 minutes**

**Servings: 4**

**Ingredients:**

- 4 frozen corn on the cob, cut in half
- ½ tsp of thyme
- 1 tbsp. of grated parmesan cheese
- ¼ tsp of black pepper

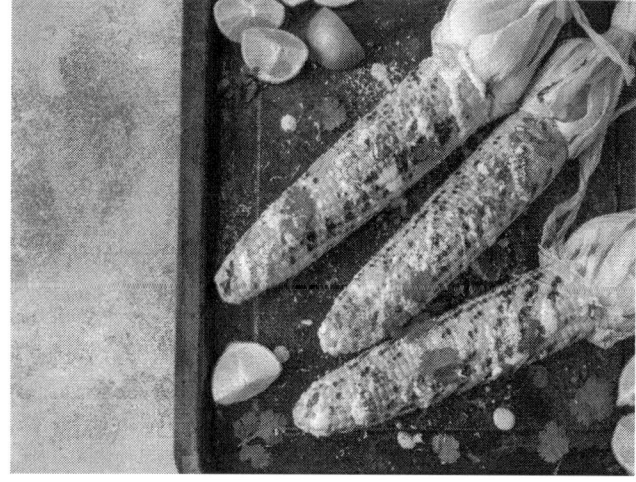

**Directions:**

1. Combine the oil, cheese, thyme, and black pepper in a bowl.
2. Place the corn in the cheese/oil mix and roll to coat evenly.
3. Fold all 4 pieces in aluminum foil, leaving a small open surface on top.
4. Place the wrapped corns over the grill and let cook for 20 minutes.
5. Serve hot.

**Nutrition:**

Calories: 125

Carbohydrate: 29.5 g

Protein: 2 g

Fat: 1.3 g

Sodium: 26 g

Potassium: 145 mg

Phosphorus: 91.5 mg

## 48. Couscous with Veggies

**Preparation Time:** 10 minutes

**Cooking Time:** 10 minutes

**Servings:** 5

**Ingredients:**

- ½ cup of uncooked couscous
- ¼ cup of white mushrooms, sliced
- ½ cup of red onion, chopped
- 1 garlic clove, minced
- ½ cup of frozen peas
- 2 tbsp. of dry white wine
- ½ tsp of basil
- 2 tbsp. of fresh parsley, chopped
- 1 cup water or vegetable stock
- 1 tbsp. of margarine or vegetable oil

**Directions:**

1. Thaw the peas by setting them aside at room temperature for 15-20 minutes.
2. In a medium pan, heat the margarine or vegetable oil.
3. Add the onions, peas, mushroom, and garlic and sauté for around 5 minutes. Add the wine and let it evaporate.
4. Add all the herbs and spices and toss well. Take off the heat and keep aside.
5. In a small pot, cook the couscous with 1 cup of hot water or vegetable stock. Bring to a boil, take off the heat, and sit for a few minutes with a lid covered.
6. Add the sauté veggies to the couscous and toss well.
7. Serve in a serving bowl warm or cold.

**Nutrition:**

Calories: 110.4

Carbohydrate: 18 g

Protein: 3 g

Fat: 2 g

Sodium: 112.2 mg

Potassium: 69.6 mg

Phosphorus: 46.8 mg

## 49. Easy Egg Salad

**Preparation Time:** 5 minutes

**Cooking Time:** 8 minutes

**Servings:** 4

**Ingredients:**

- 4 large eggs
- ½ cup of sweet onion, chopped
- ¼ cup of celery, chopped
- 1 tbsp. of yellow mustard
- 1 tsp of smoked paprika
- 3 tbsp. of mayo

**Directions:**

1. Hard boil the eggs in a small pot filled with water for approx. 7-8 minutes. Leave the eggs in the water for an extra couple of minutes before peeling.
2. Peel the eggs and chop finely with a knife or tool.
3. Combine all the chopped veggies with the mayo and mustard. Add in the eggs and mix well.
4. Sprinkle with some smoked paprika on top.
5. Serve cold with pitta, white bread slices, or lettuce wraps.

**Nutrition:**

Calories: 127

Carbohydrate: 6 g

Protein: 7 g

Fat: 13 g

Sodium: 170.7 mg

Potassium: 87.5 mg

Phosphorus: 101 mg

## 50. Cauliflower Rice and Coconut

**Preparation Time:** 20 minutes

**Cooking Time:** 20 minutes

Serving: 4

**Ingredients:**

- 3 cups cauliflower, riced
- 2/3 cups full-fat coconut milk
- 1-2 teaspoons sriracha paste
- ¼- ½ teaspoon onion powder
- Salt as needed
- Fresh basil for garnish

**Directions:**

Take a pan and place it over medium-low heat

Add all of the ingredients and stir them until fully combined

Cook for about 5-10 minutes, making sure that the lid is on

Remove the lid and keep cooking until there's no excess liquid

Once the rice is soft and creamy, enjoy it!

**Nutrition:**

Calories: 95

Fat: 7g

Carbohydrates: 4g

Protein: 1g

## 51. Kale and Garlic Platter

**Preparation Time:** 5 minutes

**Cooking Time:** 10 minutes

Serving: 4

**Ingredients:**

- 1 bunch kale
- 2 tablespoons olive oil
- 4 garlic cloves, minced

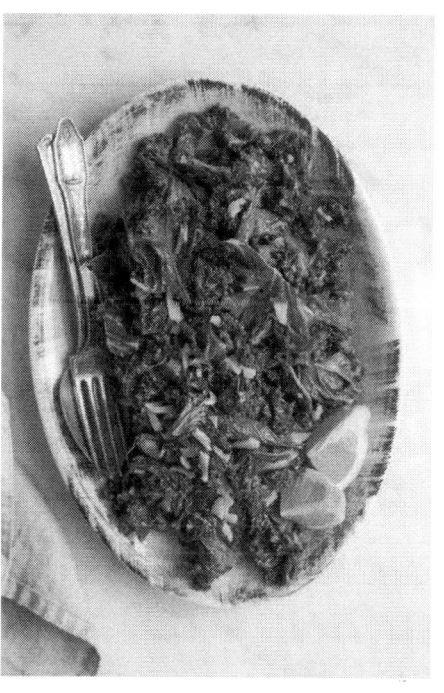

**Directions:**

- Carefully tear the kale into bite-sized portions, making sure to remove the stem
- Discard the stems
- Place on a pot over medium heat.
- Add olive oil, let heat.
- Add garlic and stir for 2 minutes
- Add kale and cook for 5-10 minutes
- Serve!

**Nutrition:**

Calories: 121

Fat: 8g

Carbohydrates: 5g

Protein: 4g

## 52. Blistered Beans and Almond

**Preparation Time:** 10 minutes

**Cooking Time:** 20 minutes

Serving: 4

**Ingredients:**

	1-pound fresh green beans, ends trimmed

	1 ½ tablespoon olive oil

	¼ teaspoon salt

	1 ½ tablespoons fresh dill, minced

	Juice of 1 lemon

	¼ cup crushed almonds

	Salt as needed

**Directions:**

	Preheat your oven to 400 °F

	Add in the green beans with your olive oil and also the salt

	Then spread them in one single layer on a large-sized sheet pan

	Roast for 10 minutes and stir nicely, then roast for another 8-10 minutes

	Remove it from the oven and keep stirring in the lemon juice alongside the dill

	Top it with crushed almonds, some flaky sea salt and serve

**Nutrition:**

Calories: 347

Fat: 16g

Carbohydrates: 6g

Protein: 45g

## 53. Cucumber Soup

**Preparation Time:** 14 minutes

**Cooking Time:** 0 minutes

Serving: 4

**Ingredients:**

- 2 tablespoons garlic, minced
- 4 cups English cucumbers, peeled and diced
- ½ cup onions, diced
- 1 tablespoon lemon juice
- 1 ½ cups vegetable broth
- ½ teaspoon salt
- ¼ teaspoon red pepper flakes
- ¼ cup parsley, diced
- ½ cup Greek yogurt, plain

**Directions:**

- Emulsify all the ingredients by blending them (except ½ cup of chopped cucumbers)
- Blend until smooth
- Divide the soup amongst 4 servings and top with extra cucumbers
- Enjoy chilled!

Nutrition

Calories: 371

Fat: 36g

Carbohydrates: 8g

Protein: 4g

## 54. Eggplant Salad

**Preparation Time:** 10 minutes

**Cooking Time:** 30 minutes

Serving: 3

**Ingredients:**

- 2 eggplants, peeled and sliced
- 2 garlic cloves
- 2 green bell paper, sliced, seeds removed
- ½ cup fresh parsley
- ½ cup egg-free mayonnaise
- Salt and black pepper

**Directions:**

- Preheat your oven to 480 °F
- Take a baking pan and add the eggplants and black pepper
- Bake for about 30 minutes
- Flip the vegetables after 20 minutes
- Then, take a bowl and add baked vegetables and all the remaining ingredients
- Mix well
- Serve and enjoy!

**Nutrition:**

Calories: 196

Fat: 108.g

Carbohydrates: 13.4g

Protein: 14.6g

## 55. Cajun Crab

**Preparation Time:** 10 minutes

**Cooking Time:** 10 minutes

Serving: 2

**Ingredients:**

1 lemon, fresh and quartered

3 tablespoons Cajun seasoning

2 bay leaves

4 snow crab legs, precooked and defrosted

Golden ghee

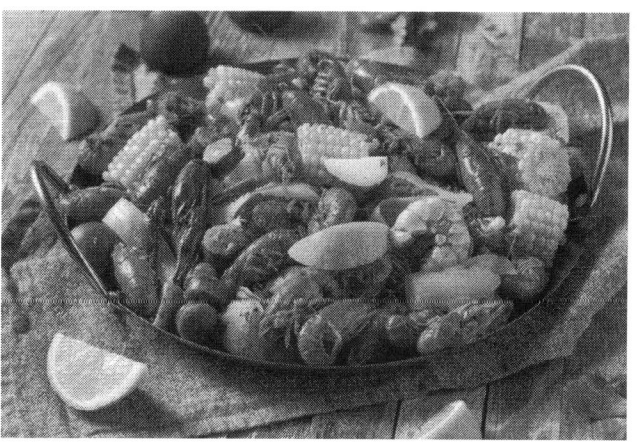

**Directions:**

Fill half large pot with salted water about.

Bring the water to a boil

Squeeze lemon juice into a pot and toss in remaining lemon quarters

Add bay leaves and Cajun seasoning

Then season for 1 minute

Add crab legs and boil for 8 minutes (make sure to keep them submerged the whole time)

Melt ghee in the microwave and use as a dipping sauce, enjoy!

Nutrition

Calories: 643

Fat: 51g

Carbohydrates: 3g

Protein: 41g

## 56. Mushroom Pork Chops

**Preparation Time:** 10 minutes
**Cooking Time:** 40 minutes
Serving: 3

**Ingredients:**

- 8 ounces mushrooms, sliced
- 1 teaspoon garlic
- 1 onion, peeled and chopped
- 1 cup egg-free mayonnaise
- 3 pork chops, boneless
- 1 teaspoon ground nutmeg
- 1 tablespoon balsamic vinegar
- ½ cup of coconut oil

**Directions:**

- Take a pan and place it over medium heat
- Add oil and let it heat up
- Add mushrooms, onions, and stir
- Cook for 4 minutes
- Add pork chops, season with nutmeg, garlic powder, and brown both sides
- Transfer the pan in the oven and bake for 30 minutes at 350 °F
- Transfer pork chops to plates and keep it warm
- Take a pan and place it over medium heat
- Add vinegar, mayonnaise over mushroom mix and stir for a few minutes
- Drizzle sauce over pork chops
- Enjoy!

**Nutrition:**

Calories: 600
Fat: 10g
Carbohydrates: 8g
Protein: 30g

## 57. Caramelized Pork Chops

**Preparation Time:** 5 minutes

**Cooking Time:** 30 minutes

Serving: 4

**Ingredients:**

- 4 pounds chuck roast
- 4 ounces green chili, chopped
- 2 tablespoons chili powder
- ½ teaspoon dried oregano
- ½ teaspoon ground cumin
- 2 garlic cloves, minced
- Salt as needed

**Directions:**

- Rub your chop with 1 teaspoon of pepper and 2 teaspoons of seasoning salt
- Take a skillet and heat some oil over medium heat
- Brown your pork chops on each side
- Add water and onions to the pan
- Simmer it for about 20 minutes
- Turn your chops over and add the rest of the pepper and salt
- Put the lid and cook until there is no water and the onions turn a medium brown texture
- Remove the chops from your pan and serve with some onions on top!

Nutrition

Calories: 271

Fat: 19g

Carbohydrates: 4g

Protein: 27g

## 58. Mediterranean Pork

**Preparation Time:** 10 minutes

**Cooking Time:** 35 minutes

Serving: 4

**Ingredients:**

- 4 pork chops, bone-in
- Salt and pepper to taste
- 1 teaspoon dried rosemary
- 3 garlic cloves, peeled and minced

**Directions:**

- Season pork chops with salt and pepper
- Place in roasting pan
- Add rosemary, garlic in a pan
- Preheat your oven to 425 ° F
- Bake for 10 minutes
- Lower heat to 350 ° F
- Roast for 25 minutes more
- Slice pork and divide on plates
- Drizzle pan juice all over
- Serve and enjoy!

**Nutrition:**

Calories: 165

Fat: 2g

Carbohydrates: 2g

Protein: 26g

## 59. Ground Beef and Bell Peppers

**Preparation Time:** 10 minutes

**Cooking Time:** 10 minutes

Serving: 3

**Ingredients:**

- 1 onion, chopped
- 2 tablespoons coconut oil
- 1-pound ground beef
- 1 red bell pepper, diced
- 2 cups green lettuce, chopped
- Salt and pepper to taste

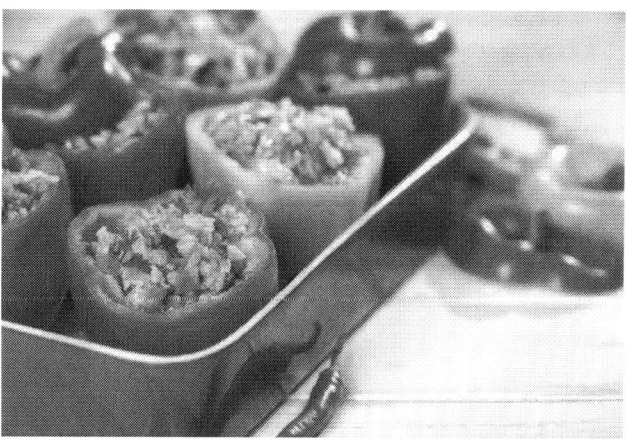

**Directions:**

- Place over medium heat on a skillet
- Add onion and cook until slightly browned
- Add green lettuce and ground beef
- Stir fry until done
- Take the mixture and fill up the bell peppers
- Serve and enjoy!

Nutrition

Calories: 350

Fat: 23g

Carbohydrates: 4g

Protein: 28g

## 60. Spiced Up Pork Chops

**Preparation Time:** 4 hours 10 minutes
**Cooking Time:** 15 minutes
Serving: 4

**Ingredients:**

- ¼ cup lime juice
- 4 pork rib chops
- 1 tablespoon coconut oil, melted
- 2 garlic cloves, peeled and minced
- 1 tablespoon chili powder
- 1 teaspoon ground cinnamon
- 2 teaspoons cumin
- Salt and pepper to taste
- ½ teaspoon hot pepper sauce
- Mango, sliced

**Directions:**

- Take a bowl and mix in lime juice, oil, garlic, cumin, cinnamon, chili powder, salt, pepper, hot pepper sauce
- Whisk well
- Add pork chops and toss
- Keep it on the side and refrigerate for 4 hours
- Pre-heat your grill to medium and transfer pork chops to a pre-heated grill
- Grill for 7 minutes both sides
- Divide between serving platters and serve with mango slices
- Enjoy!

Nutrition
Calories: 200
Fat: 8g
Carbohydrates: 3g
Protein: 26g

## 61. Juicy Salmon Dish

**Preparation Time:** 5 minutes
**Cooking Time:** 6 minutes
Serving: 3

**Ingredients:**

- ¾ cup of water
- Few sprigs of parsley, basil, tarragon, basil
- 1 pound of salmon, skin on
- 3 teaspoons of ghee
- ¼ teaspoon of salt
- ½ teaspoon of pepper
- ½ of lemon, thinly sliced
- 1 whole carrot, julienned

**Directions:**

- Set your pot to Sauté mode and add water and herbs
- Place a steamer rack inside your pot and place salmon
- Drizzle ghee on top of the salmon and season with salt and pepper
- Cover with lemon slices
- Cook on HIGH pressure with locked lid for 3 minutes
- Release the pressure naturally over 10 minutes
- Transfer the salmon to a serving platter
- Set your pot to Sauté mode and add vegetables
- Cook for 1-2 minutes
- Serve with vegetables and salmon
- Enjoy!

Nutrition Values
Calories: 464
Fat: 34g
Carbohydrates: 3g
Protein: 34g

## 62. Platter-O-Brussels

**Preparation Time:** 10 minutes

**Cooking Time:** 20 minutes

Serving: 4

**Ingredients:**

- 2 tablespoons olive oil
- 1 yellow onion, chopped
- 2 pounds Brussels sprouts, trimmed and halved
- 4 cups chicken stock
- ¼ cup coconut cream

**Directions:**

- Take a pot and place over medium heat
- Add oil and let it heat up
- Add onion and stir cook for 3 minutes
- Add Brussels sprouts and stir, cook for 2 minutes
- Add stock and black pepper, stir and bring to a simmer
- Cook for 20 minutes more
- Blend until creamy.
- Add coconut cream and stir well
- Ladle into soup bowls and serve
- Enjoy!

Nutrition

Calories: 200

Fat: 11g

Carbohydrates: 6g

Protein: 11g

## 63. Almond Chicken

**Preparation Time:** 15 minutes

**Cooking Time:** 15 minutes

Serving: 3

**Ingredients:**

- 2 large chicken breasts, boneless and skinless
- 1/3 cup lemon juice
- 1 ½ cups seasoned almond meal
- 2 tablespoons coconut oil
- Lemon pepper, to taste
- Parsley for decoration

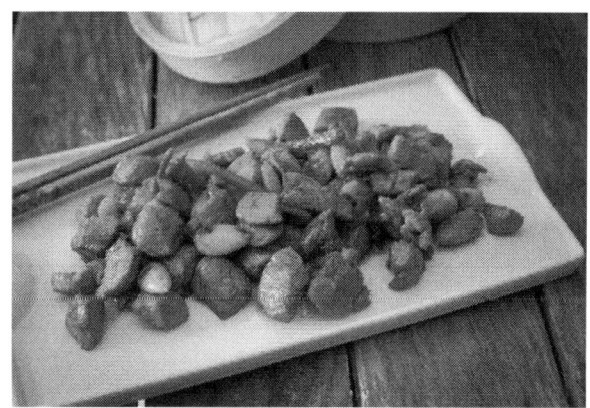

**Directions:**

- Slice chicken breast in half
- Pound out each half until ¼ inch thick
- Take a pan and place over medium heat, add oil and heat it up
- Dip each chicken breast slice into lemon juice and let it sit for 2 minutes
- Turnover and let the other side sit for 2 minutes as well
- Transfer to almond meal and coat both sides
- Add coated chicken and fry for 4 minutes per side, making sure to sprinkle lemon pepper liberally
- Transfer to a paper-lined sheet and repeat until all chicken is fried
- Garnish with parsley and enjoy!

Nutrition

Calories: 325

Fat: 24g

Carbohydrates: 3g

Protein: 16g

## 64. BlackBerry Chicken Wings

**Preparation Time:** 35 minutes

**Cooking Time:** 50 minutes

Serving: 4

**Ingredients:**

    3 pounds chicken wings, about 20 pieces

    ½ cup blackberry chipotle jam

    Salt and pepper to taste

    ½ cup of water

**Directions:**

    Add water and jam to a bowl and mix well

    Place chicken wings in a zip bag and add two-thirds of the marinade

    Season with salt and pepper

    Let it marinate for 30 minutes

    Preheat your oven to 400°F

    Prepare a baking sheet and wire rack, place chicken wings in a wire rack and bake for 15 minutes

    Brush remaining marinade and bake for 30 minutes more

    Enjoy!

Nutrition

Calories: 502

Fat: 39g

Carbohydrates: 01.8g

Protein: 34g

## 65. Aromatic Carrot Cream

**Preparation Time:** 15 minutes

**Cooking Time:** 25 minutes

**Servings:** 4

**Ingredients:**

    1 tablespoon olive oil

    ½ sweet onion, chopped

    2 teaspoons fresh ginger, peeled and grated

    1 teaspoon fresh garlic, minced

    4 cups water

    3 carrots, chopped

    1 teaspoon ground turmeric

    ½ cup coconut milk

**Directions:**

Heat the olive oil into a big pan over medium-high heat.

Add the onion, garlic and ginger. Softly cook for about 3 minutes until softened.

Include the water, turmeric and the carrots. Softly cook for about 20 minutes (until the carrots are softened).

Blend the soup adding coconut milk until creamy.

Serve and enjoy!

**Nutrition:**

Calories 112

Fat 10 g

Cholesterol 0 mg

Carbohydrates 8 g

Sugar 5 g

Fiber 2 g

Protein 2 g

Sodium 35 mg

Calcium 32 mg

Phosphorus 59 mg

Potassium 241 mg

## 66. Mushrooms Velvet Soup

**Preparation Time:** 40 minutes

**Cooking Time:** 40 minutes

**Servings:** 6

**Ingredients:**

    1 teaspoon olive oil

    ½ teaspoon fresh ground black pepper

    3 medium (85g) shallots, diced

    2 stalks (80g) celery, chopped

    1 clove garlic, diced

    12-ounces cremini mushrooms, sliced

    5 tablespoons flour

    4 cups low sodium vegetable stock, divided

    3 sprigs fresh thyme

    2 bay leaves

    ½ cup regular yogurt

**Directions:**

    Heat oil in a large pan.

    Add ground pepper, shallots and celery. Cook over medium-high heat.

    Sauté for 2 minutes until golden.

    Add garlic and stir.

    Include the sliced mushrooms. Stir and cook until the mushrooms give out their liquid.

    Sprawl the flour on the mushrooms and toast for about 2 min.

    Add one cup of hot stock, thyme sprigs and bay leaves. Stir and add the second cup of stock Stir until well combined.

    Add the remaining cups of stock.

    Slowly cook for 15 minutes.

    Take out bay leaves and thyme sprigs.

    Blend until mixture is smooth.

    Include the yogurt and stir well.

    Slowly cook for 4 minutes.

    Serve and enjoy!

**Nutrition:**

Calories 126 Fat 8 g Cholesterol 0 mg Carbohydrate 14 g Sugar 4 g

Fiber 2 g Protein 3 g Sodium 108 mg Calcium 55 mg Phosphorus 70 mg Potassium 298 mg

## 67. Easy Lettuce Wraps

**Preparation Time:** 15 minutes

**Cooking Time:** 0 minutes

**Servings:** 4

**Ingredients:**

- 8 ounces cooked chicken, shredded
- 1 scallion, chopped
- ½ cup seedless red grapes, halved
- 1 celery stalk, chopped
- ¼ cup mayonnaise
- A pinch ground black pepper
- 4 large lettuce leaves

**Directions:**

- In a mixing bowl add the scallion, chicken, celery, grapes and mayonnaise.
- Stir well until incorporated.
- Season with pepper.
- Place the lettuce leaves onto serving plates.
- Place the chicken salad onto the leaves.
- Serve and enjoy!

**Nutrition:**

Calories 146

Fat 5 g

Cholesterol 35 mg

Carbohydrates 8 g

Sugar 4 g

Fiber 0 g

Protein 16 g

Sodium 58 mg

Calcium 18 mg

Phosphorus 125 mg

Potassium 212 mg

## 68. Spaghetti with Pesto

**Preparation Time:** 10 minutes

**Cooking Time:** 10 minutes

**Servings:** 4

**Ingredients:**

- 8 ounces spaghetti (package pasta)
- 2 cups packed basil leaves
- 2 cups packed arugula leaves
- 1/3 cup walnut pieces
- 3 cloves of garlic
- ¼ cup extra-virgin olive oil
- Black pepper

**Directions:**

Cook pasta with boiling water. Drain.

Add the basil, garlic, olive oil, walnuts, pepper and arugula in a blender and mix until creamy.

Mix pesto mixture into pasta in a large bowl.

Serve and enjoy!

**Nutrition:**

Calories 400

Fat 21 g

Cholesterol 0 mg

Carbohydrates 46 g

Sugar 2 g

Fiber 3 g

Protein 11 g

Sodium 6 mg

Calcium 64 mg

Phosphorus 113 mg

Potassium 202 mg

## 69. Vegetable Casserole

**Preparation Time:** 15 minutes
**Cooking Time:** 15 minutes
**Servings:** 8
**Ingredients:**

- 1 teaspoon olive oil
- 1 sweet onion, chopped
- 1 teaspoon garlic, minced
- 2 zucchinis, chopped
- 1 red bell pepper, diced
- 2 carrots, chopped
- 2 cups low-sodium vegetable stock
- 2 large Red bell peppers, chopped
- 2 cups broccoli florets
- 1 teaspoon ground coriander
- ½ teaspoon ground comminutes
- Black pepper

**Directions:**

Heat the olive oil into a big pan over medium-high heat.

Add onion and garlic. Softly cook for about 3 minutes until softened.

Include the zucchini, carrots, bell pepper and softly cook for 5-6 minutes.

Pour the vegetable stock, Red bell peppers, broccoli, coriander, cumin, pepper and stir well.

Softly cook for about 5 minutes over medium-high heat until the vegetables are tender.

Serve hot and enjoy!

**Nutrition:**

Calories 47
Fat 1 g
Cholesterol 0 g
Carbohydrates 8 g
Sugar 6 g
Fiber 2 g
Protein 2 g
Sodium 104 mg
Calcium 36 mg Phosphorus 52 mg
Potassium 298 mg

## 70. Appetizing Rice Salad

**Preparation Time:** 20 minutes

**Cooking Time:** 1 hour

**Servings:** 8

**Ingredients:**

- 1 cup wild rice
- 2 cups water
- 1 tablespoon olive oil
- 2/3 cup walnuts, chopped
- 1 (4 inches) celery rib, sliced
- 4 scallions, thinly sliced
- 1 medium red apple, cored and diced
- ½ cup pomegranate seeds
- ½ tablespoon lemon zest
- 3 tablespoons lemon juice
- Black pepper
- 1/3 cup olive oil

**Directions:**

1. In a big pot place the wild strained rice together with water and olive oil.
2. Bring to a boil and simmer for about 50 minutes until rice is tender.
3. In a mixing bowl add celery, walnuts, apple, scallions, pomegranate seeds and lemon zest.
4. Mix well with a blender the lemon juice, pepper, and olive oil.
5. Spread half of this dressing on the apple mixture and mix well.
6. When the rice is cooked, let it cool and incorporate with the fruit mixture
7. Season with the remaining dressing.
8. Serve at room temperature and enjoy!

**Nutrition:**

Calories 300 Fat 19 g

Cholesterol 0 mg

Carbohydrates 34 g

Sugar 11 g Fiber 5 g Protein 6 g

Sodium 6 mg Calcium 30 mg

Phosphorus 144 mg

Potassium 296 mg

## 71. Spiced Wraps

**Preparation Time:** 30 minutes
**Cooking Time:** 0 minutes
**Servings:** 8
**Ingredients:**

- 6 ounces cooked chicken breast, minced
- 1 scallion, chopped
- ½ red apple, cored and chopped
- ½ cup bean sprouts
- ¼ cucumber, chopped
- Juice of 1 lime
- Zest of 1 lime
- 2 tablespoons fresh cilantro, chopped
- ½ teaspoon Chinese five-spice powder
- 8 lettuce leaves

**Directions:**

- Combine the chicken, apple, bean sprouts, cucumber, lime juice, lime zest, cilantro, five-spice powder and scallions.
- Place the lettuce leaves onto 8 serving plates.
- Spoon the chicken mixture onto lettuce leaves.
- Wrap the lettuce around the chicken mixture.
- Serve and enjoy!

**Nutrition:**

Calories 53
Fat 3 g
Cholesterol 19 mg
Carbohydrates 3 g
Sugar 3 g
Fiber 2 g
Protein 7 g
Sodium 19 mg
Calcium 16 mg
Phosphorus 58 mg
Potassium 134

## 72. Rump Roast

**Preparation Time:** 10 minutes
**Cooking Time:** 5 hours
**Servings:** 8
**Ingredients:**

- 1-pound rump roast
- ½ teaspoon black pepper
- 1 tablespoon olive oil
- ½ small onion, chopped
- 2 teaspoons garlic, minced
- 1 teaspoon dried thyme
- 1 cup + 3 tablespoons water
- 2 tablespoons cornstarch

**Directions:**

Heat the olive oil into a big saucepan over medium heat.

Add the peppered meat and brown the roast all over. Set aside the meat.

Softly cook the garlic and onion in the same saucepan for about 3 minutes until they are tendered.

Incorporate the roast to the saucepan, add 1 cup of water and the thyme.

Cover, simmer until the meat is tender or for 4 and half hours.

In a mixing bowl, stir the cornstarch with 3 tablespoons water to form a slurry.

Beat the slurry into the liquid in the pan and cook for about 15 minutes to thicken the sauce.

Serve and enjoy!

**Nutrition:**

Calories 156

Fat 12 g

Cholesterol 42 mg

Carbohydrates 4 g

Sugar 2 g

Fiber 0 g

Protein 14 g

Sodium 48 mg

Calcium 18 mg

Phosphorus 114 mg

Potassium 220 mg

# CHAPTER 7:

# Dinner

## 73. Beef Kabobs with Pepper

**Preparation Time:** 5 Minutes
**Cooking Time:** 10 Minutes
**Servings:** 8
**Ingredients:**

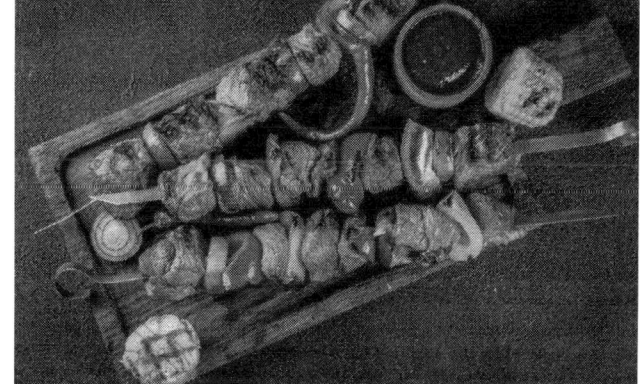

- 1 Pound of beef sirloin
- 1/2 Cup of vinegar
- 2 tbsp. of salad oil
- 1 Medium, chopped onion
- 2 tbsp. of chopped fresh parsley
- 1/4 tsp. of black pepper
- 2 Cut into strips green peppers

**Directions:**

1. Trim the fat from the meat; then cut it into cubes of 1 and 1/2 inches each
2. Mix the vinegar, the oil, the onion, the parsley and the pepper in a bowl
3. Place the meat in the marinade and set it aside for about 2 hours; make sure to stir from time to time.
4. Remove the meat from the marinade and alternate it on skewers instead with green pepper
5. Brush the pepper with the marinade and broil for about 10 minutes 4 inches from the heat
6. Serve and enjoy your kabobs

**Nutrition:**

Calories: 357 kcal
Total Fat: 24 g
Saturated Fat: 0 g
Cholesterol: 9 mg
Sodium: 60 mg
Total Carbs: 0 g

## 74. One-Pot Beef Roast

**Preparation Time:** 10 minutes

**Cooking Time:** 75 minutes

**Servings:** 4

**Ingredients:**

- 3 1/2 pounds beef roast
- 4 ounces mushrooms, sliced
- 12 ounces beef stock
- 1-ounce onion soup mix
- 1/2 cup Italian dressing

**Directions:**

1. Take a bowl and add the stock, onion soup mix, and Italian dressing
2. Stir
3. Put beef roast in pan
4. Add the mushrooms and stock mix to the pan and cover with foil
5. Preheat your oven to 300 °F
6. Bake for 1 hour and 15 minutes
7. Let the roast cool
8. Slice and serve
9. Enjoy the gravy on top!

**Nutrition:**

Calories: 700 kcal

Total Fat: 56 g

Saturated Fat: 0 g

Cholesterol: 0 mg

Sodium: 0 mg

Total Carbs: 10 g

## 75. Cabbage and Beef Fry

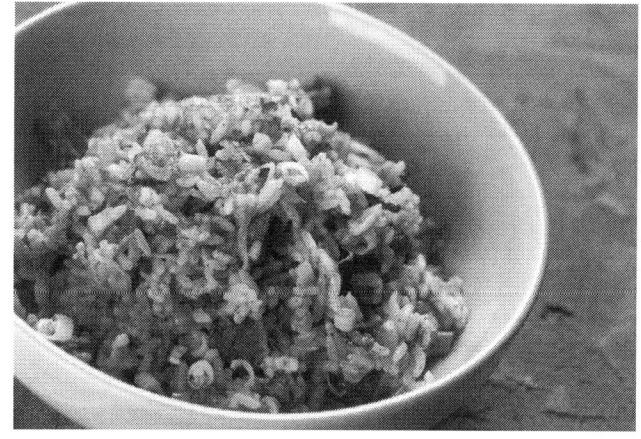

**Preparation Time:** 5 minutes

**Cooking Time:** 15 minutes

**Servings:** 4

**Ingredients:**

- 1 pound beef, ground
- 1/2 pound bacon
- 1 onion
- 1 garlic cloves, minced
- 1/2 head cabbage
- Salt and pepper to taste

**Directions:**

1. Take a skillet and place it over medium heat
2. Add chopped bacon, beef and onion until slightly browned
3. Transfer to a bowl and keep it covered
4. Add minced garlic and cabbage to the skillet and cook until slightly browned
5. Return the ground beef mixture to the skillet and simmer for 3-5 minutes over low heat
6. Serve and enjoy!

**Nutrition:**

Calories: 360 kcal

Total Fat: 22 g

Saturated Fat: 0 g

Cholesterol: 0 mg

Sodium: 0 mg

Total Carbs: 5 g

## 76. California Pork Chops

**Preparation Time:** 10 minutes

**Cooking Time:** 10 minutes

**Servings:** 2

**Ingredients:**

- 1 tbsp. fresh cilantro, chopped
- 1/2 cup chives, chopped
- 2 large green bell peppers, chopped
- 1 lb. 1" thick boneless pork chops
- 1 tbsp. fresh lime juice
- 2 cups cooked rice
- 1/8 tsp. dried oregano leaves
- 1/4 tsp. ground black pepper
- 1/4 tsp. ground cumin
- 1 tbsp. butter
- 1 lime

**Directions:**

1. Start by seasoning the pork chops with lime juice and cilantro.
2. Place them in a shallow dish.
3. Toss the chives with pepper, cumin, butter, oregano and rice in a bowl.
4. Stuff the bell peppers with this mixture and place them around the pork chops.
5. Cover the chop and bell peppers with a foil sheet and bake them for 10 minutes in the oven at 375 degrees f.
6. Serve warm.

**Nutrition:**

Calories: 265 kcal

Total Fat: 15 g

Saturated Fat: 0 g

Cholesterol: 86 mg

Sodium: 70 mg

Total Carbs: 24 g

Fiber: 1 g

Sugar: 0 g

Protein: 34 g

## 77. Caribbean Turkey Curry

**Preparation Time:** 10 minutes

**Cooking Time:** 1 hour an 30 minutes

**Servings:** 6

**Ingredients:**

- 3 1/2 lbs. turkey breast, with skin
- 1/4 cup butter, melted
- 1/4 cup honey
- 1 tbsp. mustard
- 2 tsp. curry powder
- 1 tsp. garlic powder

**Directions:**

1. Place the turkey breast in a shallow roasting pan.
2. Insert a meat thermometer to monitor the temperature.
3. Bake the turkey for 1.5 hours at 350 degrees f until its internal temperature reaches 170 degrees f.
4. Meanwhile, thoroughly mix honey, butter, curry powder, garlic powder, and mustard in a bowl.
5. Glaze the cooked turkey with this mixture liberally.
6. Let it sit for 15 minutes for absorption.
7. Slice and serve.

**Nutrition:**

Calories: 275 kcal

Total Fat: 13 g

Saturated Fat: 0 g

Cholesterol: 82 mg

Sodium: 122 mg

Total Carbs: 90 g

## 78. Chicken Fajitas

**Preparation Time:** 10 minutes

**Cooking Time:** 10 minutes

**Servings:** 8

**Ingredients:**

- 8 flour tortillas, 6" size
- 1/4 cup green pepper, cut in strips
- 1/4 cup red pepper, cut in strips
- 1/2 cup onion, sliced
- 1/2 cup cilantro
- 2 tbsp. canola oil
- 12 oz. boneless chicken breasts
- 1/4 tsp. black pepper
- 2 tsp. chili powder
- 1/2 tsp. cumin
- 2 tbsp. lemon juice

**Directions:**

1. Start by wrapping the tortillas in a foil.
2. Warm them up for 10 minutes in a preheated oven at 300 degrees f.
3. Add oil to a nonstick pan.
4. Add lemon juice chicken and seasoning
5. Stir fry for 5 minutes then add onion and peppers.
6. Continue cooking for 5 minutes or until chicken is tender.
7. Stir in cilantro, mix well and serve in tortillas.

**Nutrition:**

Calories: 343 kcal

Total Fat: 13 g

Saturated Fat: 0 g

Cholesterol: 53 mg

Sodium: 281 mg

Total Carbs: 33 g

## 79. Chicken Veronique

**Preparation Time:** 10 minutes

**Cooking Time:** 10 minutes

**Servings:** 4

**Ingredients:**

- 2 boneless skinless chicken breasts
- 1/2 shallot, chopped
- 2 tablespoons butter
- 2 tablespoons dry white wine
- 2 tablespoons chicken broth
- 1/2 cup green grapes, halved
- 1 teaspoon dried tarragon
- 1/4 cup cream

**Directions:**

1. Place an 8-inch skillet over medium heat and add butter to melt.
2. Sear the chicken in the melted butter until golden-brown on both sides.
3. Place the boneless chicken on a plate and set it aside.
4. Add shallot to the same skillet and stir until soft.
5. Whisk cornstarch with broth and wine in a small bowl.
6. Pour this slurry into the skillet and mix well.
7. Place the chicken in the skillet and cook it on a simmer for 6 minutes.
8. Transfer the chicken to the serving plate.
9. Add cream, tarragon, and grapes.
10. Cook for 1 minute, and then pour this sauce over the chicken.
11. Serve.

**Nutrition:**

Calories: 306 kcal

Total Fat: 18 g

Saturated Fat: 0 g

Cholesterol: 124 mg

Sodium: 167 mg

Total Carbs: 9 g

## 80. Chicken and Apple Curry

**Preparation Time:** 10 minutes

**Cooking Time:** 1 hour and 11 minutes

**Servings:** 8

**Ingredients:**

- 8 boneless skinless chicken breasts
- 1/4 teaspoon black pepper
- 2 medium apples, peeled, cored, and chopped
- 2 small onions, chopped
- 1 garlic clove, minced
- 3 tablespoons butter
- 1 tablespoon curry powder
- 1/2 tablespoon dried basil
- 3 tablespoons flour
- 1 cup chicken broth
- 1 cup of rice milk

**Directions:**

1. Preheat oven to 350°F.
2. Set the chicken breasts in a baking pan and sprinkle black pepper over it.
3. Place a suitably-sized saucepan over medium heat and add butter to melt.
4. Add onion, garlic, and apple, then sauté until soft.
5. Stir in basil and curry powder, and then cook for 1 minute.
6. Add flour and continue mixing for 1 minute.
7. Stir in rice milk and chicken broth, then stir cook for 5 minutes.
8. Pour this sauce over the chicken breasts in the baking pan.
9. Bake the chicken for 60 minutes then serve.

**Nutrition:**

Calories: 232 kcal

Total Fat: 8 g

Saturated Fat: 0 g

Cholesterol: 85 mg

Sodium: 118 mg

Total Carbs: 11 g

## 81. London Broil

**Preparation Time:** 10 minutes

**Cooking Time:** 5 minutes

**Servings:** 4

**Ingredients:**

- 2 pounds flank steak
- 1/4 teaspoon meat tenderizer
- 1 tablespoon sugar
- 2 tablespoons lemon juice
- 2 tablespoons soy sauce
- 1 tablespoon honey
- 1 teaspoon herb seasoning blend

**Directions:**

1. Pound the meat with a mallet then place it in a shallow dish.
2. Sprinkle meat tenderizer over the meat.
3. Whisk rest of the ingredients and spread this marinade over the meat.
4. Marinate the meat for 4 hours in the refrigerator.
5. Bake the meat for 5 minutes per side at 350°F.
6. Slice and serve.

**Nutrition:**

Calories: 184 kcal

Total Fat: 8 g

Saturated Fat: 0 g

Cholesterol: 43 mg

Sodium: 208 mg

Total Carbs: 3 g

## 82. Sirloin with Squash and Pineapple

**Preparation Time:** 10 minutes

**Cooking Time:** 9 minutes

**Servings:** 2

**Ingredients:**

- 8 ounces canned pineapple slices
- 2 garlic cloves, minced
- 2 teaspoons ginger root, minced
- 3 teaspoons olive oil
- 1 pound sirloin tips
- 1 medium zucchini, diced
- 1 medium yellow squash, diced
- 1/2 medium red onion, diced

**Directions:**

1. Mix pineapple juice with 1 teaspoon olive oil, ginger, and garlic in a Ziplock bag.
2. Add sirloin tips to the pineapple juice marinade and seal the bag.
3. Place the bag in the refrigerator overnight.
4. Preheat oven to 450°F.
5. Layer 2 sheet pans with foil and grease it with 1 teaspoon olive oil.
6. Spread the squash, onion, and pineapple rings in the prepared pans.
7. Bake them for 5 minutes then transfer to the serving plate.
8. Place the marinated sirloin tips on a baking sheet and bake for 4 minutes in the oven.
9. Transfer the sirloin tips to the roasted vegetables.
10. Serve.

**Nutrition:**

Calories: 264 kcal

Total Fat: 12 g

Saturated Fat: 0 g

Cholesterol: 74 mg

Sodium: 150 mg

Total Carbs: 14 g

## 83. Slow-Cooked BBQ Beef

**Preparation Time:** 10 minutes

**Cooking Time:** 30 minutes

**Servings:** 4

**Ingredients:**

- 4-pound pot roast
- 2 cups of water
- ¾ cup ketchup
- 1/4 cup brown sugar
- 1/3 cup vinegar
- 1/2 teaspoon allspice
- 1/4 cup onion

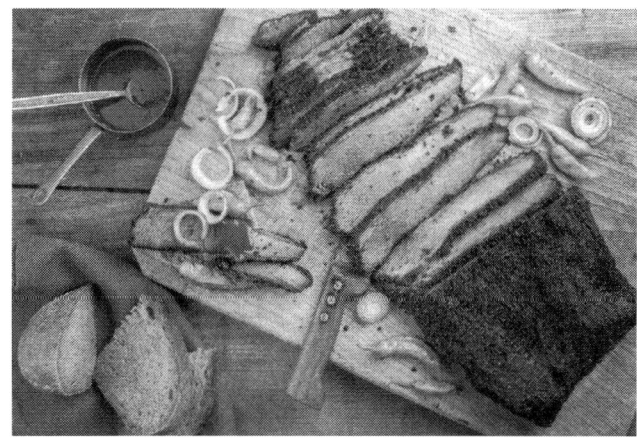

**Directions:**

1. Add 2 cups water and roast to a Crockpot and cover it.
2. Cook for 10 hours on LOW setting, then drain it while keeping 1 cup of its liquid.
3. Transfer the cooked meat to a 9x13 pan and set it aside.
4. Whisk 1 cup liquid, ketchup, vinegar, brown sugar, minced onion, and allspice in a bowl.
5. Add beef to the marinade and mix well to coat, then marinate overnight in the refrigerator.
6. Spread it on a baking pan then bake for 30 minutes at 350°F.
7. Serve.

**Nutrition:**

Calories: 303 kcal

Total Fat: 17 g

Saturated Fat: 0 g

Cholesterol: 71 mg

Sodium: 207 mg

Total Carbs: 7 g

## 84. Lemon Sprouts

**Preparation Time:** 10 minutes

**Cooking Time:** 0

**Servings:** 4

**Ingredients:**

- 1 pound Brussels sprouts, trimmed and shredded
- 8 tablespoons olive oil
- 1 lemon, juiced and zested
- Salt and pepper to taste
- ¾ cup spicy almond and seed mix

**Directions:**

1. Take a bowl and mix in lemon juice, salt, pepper and olive oil
2. Mix well
3. Stir in shredded Brussels sprouts and toss
4. Let it sit for 10 minutes
5. Add nuts and toss
6. Serve and enjoy!

**Nutrition:**

Calories: 382

Fat: 36g

Carbohydrates: 9g

Protein: 7g

## 85. Lemon and Broccoli Platter

**Preparation Time:** 10 minutes

**Cooking Time:** 15 minutes

**Servings:** 6

**Ingredients:**

- 2 heads broccoli, separated into florets
- 2 teaspoons extra virgin olive oil
- 1 teaspoon salt
- 1/2 teaspoon black pepper
- 1 garlic clove, minced
- 1/2 teaspoon lemon juice

**Directions:**

1. Preheat your oven to 400 °F
2. Take a large-sized bowl and add broccoli florets
3. Drizzle olive oil and season with pepper, salt, and garlic
4. Spread the broccoli out in a single even layer on a baking sheet
5. Bake for 15-20 minutes until fork tender
6. Squeeze lemon juice on top
7. Serve and enjoy!

**Nutrition:**

Calories: 49

Fat: 1.9g

Carbohydrates: 7g

Protein: 3g

## 86. Chicken Liver Stew

**Preparation Time:** 10 minutes

**Cooking Time:** 20 minutes

**Servings:** 2

**Ingredients:**

- 10 ounces chicken livers
- 1-ounce onion, chopped
- 2 ounces sour cream
- 1 tablespoon olive oil
- Salt to taste

**Directions:**

1. Take a pan and place it over medium heat
2. Add oil and let it heat up
3. Add onions and fry until just browned
4. Add livers and season with salt
5. Cook until livers are half cooked
6. Transfer the mix to a stew pot
7. Add sour cream and cook for 20 minutes
8. Serve and enjoy!

**Nutrition:**

Calories: 146

Fat: 9g

Carbohydrates: 2g

Protein: 15g

## 87. Simple Lamb Chops

**Preparation Time:** 35 minutes

**Cooking Time:** 5 minutes

**Servings:** 3

**Ingredients:**

- 1/4 cup olive oil
- 1/4 cup mint, fresh and chopped
- 8 lamb rib chops
- 1 tablespoon garlic, minced
- 1 tablespoon rosemary, fresh and chopped

**Directions:**

1. Add rosemary, garlic, mint, olive oil into a bowl and mix well
2. Keep a tablespoon of the mixture on the side for later use
3. Toss lamb chops into the marinade, letting them marinate for 30 minutes
4. Take a cast-iron skillet and place it over medium-high heat
5. Add lamb and cook for 2 minutes per side for medium-rare
6. Let the lamb rest for a few minutes and drizzle the remaining marinade
7. Serve and enjoy!

**Nutrition:**

Calories: 566

Fat: 40g

Carbohydrates: 2g

Protein: 47g

## 88. Chicken and Mushroom Stew

**Preparation Time:** 10 minutes

**Cooking Time:** 35 minutes

**Servings:** 4

**Ingredients:**

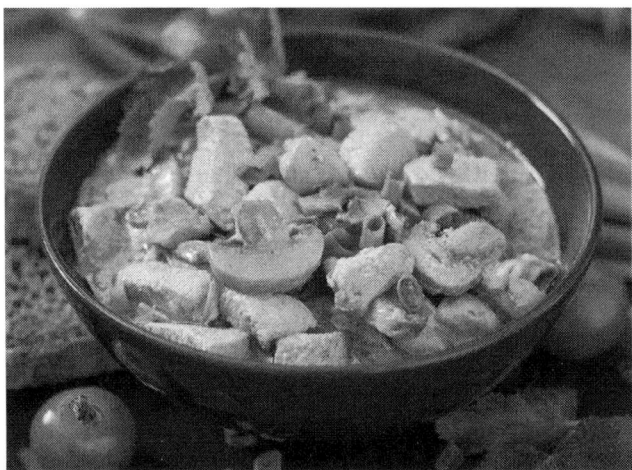

- 4 chicken breast halves, cut into bite-sized pieces
- 1 pound mushrooms, sliced (5-6 cups)
- 1 bunch spring onion, chopped
- 4 tablespoons olive oil
- 1 teaspoon thyme
- Salt and pepper as needed

**Directions:**

1. Take a large deep frying pan and place it over medium-high heat
2. Add oil and let it heat up
3. Add chicken and cook for 4-5 minutes per side until slightly browned
4. Add spring onions and mushrooms, season with salt and pepper according to your taste
5. Stir
6. Cover with lid and bring the mix to a boil
7. Lower heat and simmer for 25 minutes
8. Serve!

**Nutrition:**

Calories: 247

Fat: 12g

Carbohydrates: 10g

Protein: 23g

## 89. Roasted Carrot Soup

**Preparation Time:** 10 minutes

**Cooking Time:** 50 minutes

**Servings:** 4

**Ingredients:**

- 8 large carrots, washed and peeled
- 6 tablespoons olive oil
- 1-quart broth
- Cayenne pepper to taste
- Salt and pepper to taste

**Directions:**

1. Preheat your oven to 425 °F
2. Take a baking sheet and add carrots, drizzle olive oil and roast for 30-45 minutes
3. Put roasted carrots into a blender and add the broth, puree
4. Pour into saucepan and heat soup
5. Season with salt, pepper, and cayenne
6. Drizzle olive oil
7. Serve and enjoy!

**Nutrition:**

Calories: 222

Fat: 18g

Net Carbohydrates: 7g

Protein: 5g

## 90. Garlic and Butter-Flavored Cod

**Preparation Time:** 5 minutes
**Cooking Time:** 20 minutes
**Servings:** 3
**Ingredients:**

- 3 Cod fillets, 8 ounces each
- ¾ pound baby bok choy halved
- 1/3 cup almond butter, thinly sliced
- 1 1/2 tablespoons garlic, minced
- Salt and pepper to taste

**Directions:**

1. Preheat your oven to 400 °F
2. Cut 3 sheets of aluminum foil (large enough to fit fillet)
3. Place cod fillet on each sheet and add butter and garlic on top
4. Add bok choy, season with pepper and salt
5. Fold packet and enclose them in pouches
6. Arrange on baking sheet
7. Bake for 20 minutes
8. Transfer to a cooling rack and let them cool
9. Enjoy!

**Nutrition:**

Calories: 355

Fat: 21g

Carbohydrates: 3g

Protein: 37g

## 91. Tilapia Broccoli Platter

**Preparation Time:** 4 minutes

**Cooking Time:** 14 minutes

**Servings:** 2

**Ingredients:**

- 6 ounces of tilapia, frozen
- 1 tablespoon of almond butter
- 1 tablespoon of garlic, minced
- 1 teaspoon of lemon pepper seasoning
- 1 cup of broccoli florets, fresh

**Directions:**

1. Preheat your oven to 350 °F
2. Add fish in aluminum foil packets
3. Arrange the broccoli around fish
4. Sprinkle lemon pepper on top
5. Close the packets and seal
6. Bake for 14 minutes
7. Take a bowl and add garlic and butter, mix well and keep the mixture on the side
8. Remove the packet from the oven and transfer to a platter
9. Place butter on top of the fish and broccoli, serve and enjoy!

**Nutrition:**

Calories: 362

Fat: 25g

Carbohydrates: 2g

Protein: 29g

## 92. Parsley Scallops

**Preparation Time:** 5 minutes
**Cooking Time:** 25 minutes
**Servings:** 4

**Ingredients:**

- 8 tablespoons almond butter
- 2 garlic cloves, minced
- 16 large sea scallops
- Salt and pepper to taste
- 1 1/2 tablespoons olive oil

**Directions:**

1. Seasons scallops with salt and pepper
2. Take a skillet and place it over medium heat, add oil and let it heat up
3. Sauté scallops for 2 minutes per side, repeat until all scallops are cooked
4. Add butter to the skillet and let it melt
5. Stir in garlic and cook for 15 minutes
6. Return scallops to skillet and stir to coat
7. Serve and enjoy!

**Nutrition:**

Calories: 417
Fat: 31g
Net Carbohydrates: 5g
Protein: 29g

## 93. Blackened Chicken

**Preparation Time:** 10 minutes

**Cooking Time:** 10 minutes

**Servings:** 4

**Ingredients:**

- 1/2 teaspoon paprika
- 1/8 teaspoon salt
- 1/4 teaspoon cayenne pepper
- 1/4 teaspoon ground cumin
- 1/4 teaspoon dried thyme
- 1/8 teaspoon ground white pepper
- 1/8 teaspoon onion powder
- 2 chicken breasts, boneless and skinless

**Directions:**

1. Preheat your oven to 350 °F
2. Grease baking sheet
3. Take a cast-iron skillet and place it over high heat
4. Add oil and heat it up for 5 minutes until smoking hot
5. Take a small bowl and mix salt, paprika, cumin, white pepper, cayenne, thyme, onion powder
6. Oil the chicken breast on both sides and coat the breast with the spice mix
7. Transfer to your hot pan and cook for 1 minute per side
8. Transfer to your prepared baking sheet and bake for 5 minutes
9. Serve and enjoy!

**Nutrition:**

Calories: 136

Fat: 3g

Carbohydrates: 1g

Protein: 24g

## 94. Spicy Paprika Lamb Chops

**Preparation Time:** 10 minutes

**Cooking Time:** 15 minutes

**Servings:** 4

**Ingredients:**

- 2 lamb racks, cut into chops
- Salt and pepper to taste
- 3 tablespoons paprika
- ¾ cup cumin powder
- 1 teaspoon chili powder

**Directions:**

1. Take a bowl and add the paprika, cumin, chili, salt, pepper, and stir
2. Add lamb chops and rub the mixture
3. Heat grill over medium-temperature and add lamb chops, cook for 5 minutes
4. Flip and cook for 5 minutes more, flip again
5. Cook for 2 minutes, flip and cook for 2 minutes more
6. Serve and enjoy!

**Nutrition:**

Calories: 200

Fat: 5g

Carbohydrates: 4g

Protein: 8g

## 95. Mushroom and Olive Sirloin Steak

**Preparation Time:** 10 minutes

**Cooking Time:** 14 minutes

**Servings:** 4

**Ingredients:**

- 1 pound boneless beef sirloin steak, ¾ inch thick, cut into 4 pieces
- 1 large red onion, chopped
- 1 cup mushrooms
- 4 garlic cloves, thinly sliced
- 4 tablespoons olive oil
- 1 cup parsley leaves, finely cut

**Directions:**

1. Take a large-sized skillet and place it over medium-high heat
2. Add oil and let it heat up
3. Add beef and cook until both sides are browned, remove beef and drain fat
4. Add the rest of the oil to skillet and heat it up
5. Add onions, garlic and cook for 2-3 minutes
6. Stir well
7. Return beef to skillet and lower heat to medium
8. Cook for 3-4 minutes (covered)
9. Stir in parsley
10. Serve and enjoy!

**Nutrition:**

Calories: 386

Fat: 30g

Carbohydrates: 11g

Protein: 21g

## 96. Parsley and Chicken Breast

**Preparation Time:** 10 minutes
**Cooking Time:** 40 minutes
**Servings:** 4
**Ingredients:**

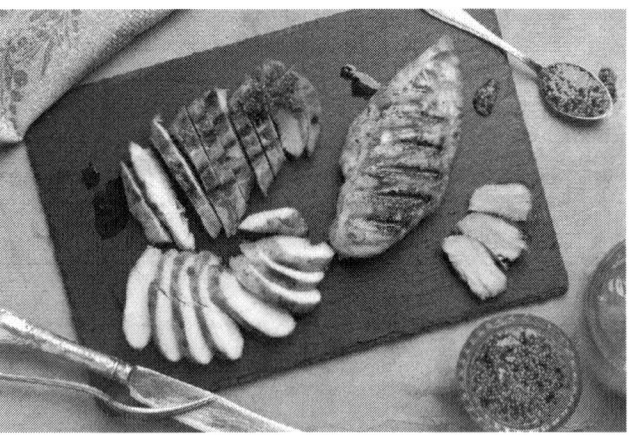

- 1 tablespoon dry parsley
- 1 tablespoon dry basil
- 4 chicken breast halves, boneless and skinless
- 1/2 teaspoon salt
- 1/2 teaspoon red pepper flakes, crushed

**Directions:**

1. Preheat your oven to 350 °F
2. Take a 9x13 inch baking dish and grease it with cooking spray
3. Sprinkle 1 tablespoon of parsley, 1 teaspoon of basil and spread the mixture over your baking dish
4. Arrange the chicken breast halves over the dish and sprinkle garlic slices on top
5. Take a small bowl and add 1 teaspoon parsley, 1 teaspoon of basil, salt, basil, red pepper and mix well. Pour the mixture over the chicken breast
6. Bake for 25 minutes
7. Remove the cover and bake for 15 minutes more
8. Serve and enjoy!

**Nutrition:**

- Calories: 150
- Fat: 4g
- Carbohydrates: 4g
- Protein: 25g

## 97. Simple Mustard Chicken

**Preparation Time:** 10 minutes

**Cooking Time:** 40 minutes

**Servings:** 4

**Ingredients:**

- 4 chicken breasts
- 1/2 cup chicken broth
- 3-4 tablespoons mustard
- 3 tablespoons olive oil
- 1 teaspoon paprika
- 1 teaspoon chili powder
- 1 teaspoon garlic powder

**Directions:**

1. Take a small bowl and mix mustard, olive oil, paprika, chicken broth, garlic powder, chicken broth, and chili
2. Add chicken breast and marinate for 30 minutes
3. Take a lined baking sheet and arrange the chicken
4. Bake for 35 minutes at 375 °F
5. Serve and enjoy!

**Nutrition:**

Calories: 531

Fat: 23g

Carbohydrates: 10g

Protein: 64g

## 98. Golden Eggplant Fries

**Preparation Time:** 10 minutes
**Cooking Time:** 15 minutes
**Servings:** 8
**Ingredients:**

- 2 eggs
- 2 cups almond flour
- 2 tablespoons coconut oil, spray
- 2 eggplant, peeled and cut thinly
- Sunflower seeds and pepper

**Directions:**

1. Preheat your oven to 400 degrees F.
2. Take a bowl and mix with sunflower seeds and black pepper.
3. Take another bowl and beat eggs until frothy.
4. Dip the eggplant pieces into the eggs.
5. Then coat them with the flour mixture.
6. Add another layer of flour and egg.
7. Then, take a baking sheet and grease with coconut oil on top.
8. Bake for about 15 minutes.
9. Serve and enjoy!

**Nutrition:** Calories: 212 Fat: 15.8g Carbohydrates: 12.1g Protein: 8.6g Phosphorus: 150mg Potassium: 147mg Sodium: 105mg

## 99. Very Wild Mushroom Pilaf

**Preparation Time:** 10 minutes

**Cooking Time:** 3 hours

**Servings:** 4

**Ingredients:**

- 1 cup wild rice
- 2 garlic cloves, minced
- 6 green onions, chopped
- 2 tablespoons olive oil
- ½ pound baby Bella mushrooms
- 2 cups water

**Directions:**

1. Add rice, garlic, onion, oil, mushrooms and water to your Slow Cooker.
2. Stir well until mixed.
3. Place lid and cook on LOW for 3 hours.
4. Stir pilaf and divide between serving platters.
5. Enjoy!

**Nutrition:** Calories: 210 Fat: 7g Carbohydrates: 16g Protein: 4g Phosphorus: 110mg Potassium: 117mg Sodium: 75mg

## 100. Sporty Baby Carrots

**Preparation Time:** 5 minutes

**Cooking Time:** 5 minutes

**Servings:** 4

**Ingredients:**

- 1-pound baby carrots
- 1 cup water
- 1 tablespoon clarified ghee
- 1 tablespoon chopped up fresh mint leaves
- Sea flavored vinegar as needed

**Directions:**

1. Place a steamer rack on top of your pot and add the carrots.
2. Add water.
3. Lock the lid and cook at HIGH pressure for 2 minutes.
4. Do a quick release.
5. Pass the carrots through a strainer and drain them.
6. Wipe the insert clean.
7. Return the insert to the pot and set the pot to Sauté mode.
8. Add clarified butter and allow it to melt.
9. Add mint and sauté for 30 seconds.
10. Add carrots to the insert and sauté well.
11. Remove them and sprinkle with bit of flavored vinegar on top.
12. Enjoy!

**Nutrition:** Calories: 131 Fat: 10g Carbohydrates: 11g Protein: 1g Phosphorus: 130mg Potassium: 147mg Sodium: 85mg

## 101. Saucy Garlic Greens

**Preparation Time:** 5 minutes

**Cooking Time:** 20 minutes

**Servings:** 4

**Ingredients:**

- 1 bunch of leafy greens
- Sauce
- ½ cup cashews soaked in water for 10 minutes
- ¼ cup water
- 1 tablespoon lemon juice
- 1 teaspoon coconut aminos
- 1 clove peeled whole clove
- 1/8 teaspoon of flavored vinegar

**Directions:**

1. Make the sauce by draining and discarding the soaking water from your cashews and add the cashews to a blender.
2. Add fresh water, lemon juice, flavored vinegar, coconut aminos, and garlic.
3. Blitz until you have a smooth cream and transfer to bowl.
4. Add ½ cup of water to the pot.
5. Place the steamer basket to the pot and add the greens in the basket.
6. Lock the lid and steam for 1 minute.
7. Quick-release the pressure.
8. Transfer the steamed greens to strainer and extract excess water.
9. Place the greens into a mixing bowl.
10. Add lemon garlic sauce and toss.
11. Enjoy!

**Nutrition:** Calories: 77 Fat: 5g Carbohydrates: 0g Protein: 2g Phosphorus: 120mg Potassium: 137mg Sodium: 85mg

## 102. Garden Salad

**Preparation Time:** 5 minutes

**Cooking Time:** 20 minutes

**Servings:** 6

**Ingredients:**

- 1-pound raw peanuts in shell
- 1 bay leaf
- 2 medium-sized chopped up Red bell peppers
- ½ cup diced up green pepper
- ½ cup diced up sweet onion
- ¼ cup finely diced hot pepper
- ¼ cup diced up celery
- 2 tablespoons olive oil
- ¾ teaspoon flavored vinegar
- ¼ teaspoon freshly ground black pepper

**Directions:**

1. Boil your peanuts for 1 minute and rinse them.
2. The skin will be soft, so discard the skin.
3. Add 2 cups of water to the Instant Pot.
4. Add bay leaf and peanuts.
5. Lock the lid and cook on HIGH pressure for 20 minutes.
6. Drain the water.
7. Take a large bowl and add the peanuts, diced up vegetables.
8. Whisk in olive oil, lemon juice, pepper in another bowl.
9. Pour the mixture over the salad and mix.
10. Enjoy!

**Nutrition:** Calories: 140 Fat: 4g Carbohydrates: 24g Protein: 5g Phosphorus: 110mg Potassium: 117mg Sodium: 75mg

## 103. Spicy Cabbage Dish

**Preparation Time:** 10 minutes

**Cooking Time:** 4 hours

**Servings:** 4

**Ingredients:**

- 2 yellow onions, chopped
- 10 cups red cabbage, shredded
- 1 cup plums, pitted and chopped
- 1 teaspoon cinnamon powder
- 1 garlic clove, minced
- 1 teaspoon cumin seeds
- ¼ teaspoon cloves, ground
- 2 tablespoons red wine vinegar
- 1 teaspoon coriander seeds
- ½ cup water

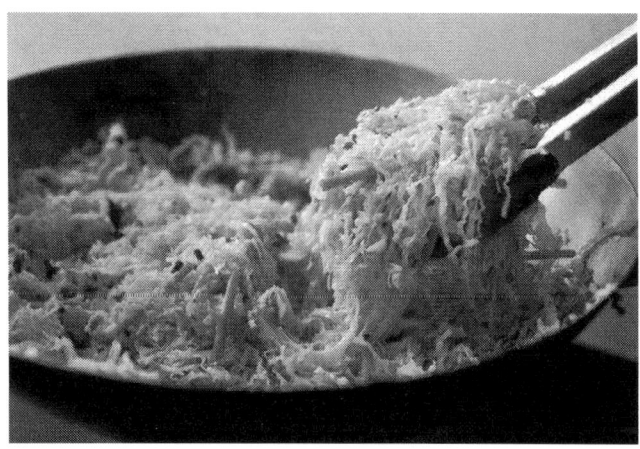

**Directions:**

1. Add cabbage, onion, plums, garlic, cumin, cinnamon, cloves, vinegar, coriander and water to your Slow Cooker.
2. Stir well.
3. Place lid and cook on LOW for 4 hours.
4. Divide between serving platters.
5. Enjoy!

**Nutrition:** Calories: 197 Fat: 1g Carbohydrates: 14g Protein: 3g Phosphorus: 115mg Potassium: 119mg Sodium: 75mg

## 104. Extreme Balsamic Chicken

**Preparation Time:** 10 minutes

**Cooking Time:** 35 minutes

**Servings:** 4

**Ingredients:**

- 3 boneless chicken breasts, skinless
- Sunflower seeds to taste
- ¼ cup almond flour
- 2/3 cups low-fat chicken broth
- 1 ½ teaspoons arrowroot
- ½ cup low sugar raspberry preserve
- 1 ½ tablespoons balsamic vinegar

**Directions:**

1. Cut chicken breast into bite-sized pieces and season them with seeds.
2. Dredge the chicken pieces in flour and shake off any excess.
3. Take a non-stick skillet and place it over medium heat.
4. Add chicken to the skillet and cook for 15 minutes, making sure to turn them half-way through.
5. Remove chicken and transfer to platter.
6. Add arrowroot, broth, raspberry preserve to the skillet and stir.
7. Stir in balsamic vinegar and reduce heat to low, stir-cook for a few minutes.
8. Transfer the chicken back to the sauce and cook for 15 minutes more.
9. Serve and enjoy!

**Nutrition:** Calories: 546 Fat: 35g Carbohydrates: 11g Protein: 44g Phosphorus: 120mg Potassium: 117mg Sodium: 85mg

## 105. Enjoyable Green lettuce and Bean Medley

**Servings:** 4

**Preparation Time:** 10 minutes

**Cooking Time:** 4 hours

**Ingredients:**

- 5 carrots, sliced
- 1 ½ cups great northern beans, dried
- 2 garlic cloves, minced
- 1 yellow onion, chopped
- Pepper to taste
- ½ teaspoon oregano, dried
- 5 ounces baby green lettuce
- 4 ½ cups low sodium veggie stock
- 2 teaspoons lemon peel, grated
- 3 tablespoon lemon juice

**Directions:**

1. Add beans, onion, carrots, garlic, oregano and stock to your Slow Cooker.
2. Stir well.
3. Place lid and cook on HIGH for 4 hours.
4. Add green lettuce, lemon juice and lemon peel.
5. Stir and let it sit for 5 minutes.
6. Divide between serving platters and enjoy!

**Nutrition:** Calories: 219 Fat: 8g Carbohydrates: 14g Protein: 8g Phosphorus: 210mg Potassium: 217mg Sodium: 85mg

## 106. Tantalizing Cauliflower and Dill Mash

**Preparation Time:** 10 minutes

**Cooking Time:** 6 hours

**Servings:** 6

**Ingredients:**

- 1 cauliflower head, florets separated
- 1/3 cup dill, chopped
- 6 garlic cloves
- 2 tablespoons olive oil
- Pinch of black pepper

**Directions:**

1. Add cauliflower to Slow Cooker.
2. Add dill, garlic and water to cover them.
3. Place lid and cook on HIGH for 5 hours.
4. Drain the flowers.
5. Season with pepper and add oil, mash using potato masher.
6. Whisk and serve.
7. Enjoy!

**Nutrition:** Calories: 207 Fat: 4g Carbohydrates: 14g Protein: 3g Phosphorus: 130mg Potassium: 107mg Sodium: 105mg

## 107. Peas Soup

**Preparation Time:** 10 minutes
**Cooking Time:** 10 minutes
**Servings:** 4
**Ingredients:**

- 1 white onion, chopped
- 1 quart veggie stock
- 2 eggs
- 3 tablespoons lemon juice
- 2 cups peas
- 2 tablespoons parmesan, grated
- Salt and black pepper to the taste

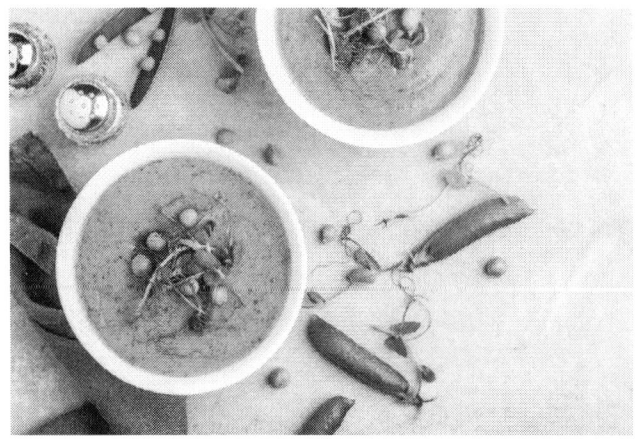

**Directions:**

1. Heat up a pot with the oil over medium-high heat, add the onion and sauté for 4 minutes.
2. Add the rest of the ingredients except the eggs, bring to a simmer and cook for 4 minutes.
3. Add whisked eggs, stir the soup, cook for 2 minutes more, divide into bowls and serve.

**Nutrition:** Calories 293, fat 11.2 fiber 3.4, carbs 27, protein 4.45

## 108. Minty Lamb Stew

**Preparation Time:** 10 minutes

**Cooking Time:** 1 hour and 45 minutes

**Servings:** 4

**Ingredients:**

- ½ cup mint, chopped
- Salt and black pepper to the taste
- 2 pounds lamb shoulder, boneless and cubed
- 3 tablespoons oil
- 1 carrot, chopped
- 1 yellow onion, chopped
- 1 celery rib, chopped
- 1 tablespoon ginger, grated
- 1 tablespoon garlic, minced
- ½ cup mint, chopped
- 15 ounces canned chickpeas, drained
- 6 tablespoons Greek yogurt

**Directions:**

1. Heat up a pot with 2 tablespoons oil over medium-high heat, add the meat and brown for 5 minutes.
2. Add the carrot, onion, celery, garlic and the ginger, stir and sauté for 5 minutes more.
3. Add the rest of the ingredients except the yogurt, bring to a simmer and cook over medium heat for 1 hour and 30 minutes.
4. Divide the stew into bowls, top each serving with the yogurt and serve.

**Nutrition:** Calories 355, fat 14.3, fiber 6.7, carbs 22.6, protein 15.4

## 109. Spicy Mushroom Stir-Fry

**Preparation Time: 10 minutes**

**Cooking Time: 10 minutes**

Servings: 4

**Ingredients:**
- 1 cup low-sodium vegetable broth
- 2 tablespoons cornstarch
- 1 teaspoon low-sodium soy sauce
- 1/2 teaspoon ground ginger
- 1/8 teaspoon cayenne pepper
- 2 tablespoons olive oil
- 2 (8-ounce) packages sliced button mushrooms
- 1 red bell pepper, chopped
- 1 jalapeño pepper, minced
- 2 tablespoons sesame oil

**Directions:**
1. In a small bowl, whisk together the broth, cornstarch, soy sauce, ginger, and cayenne pepper and set aside.
2. Heat the olive oil in a wok or heavy skillet over high heat.
3. Add the mushrooms and peppers and stir-fry for 3 to 5 minutes or until the vegetables are tender-crisp.
4. Stir the broth mixture and add it to the wok; stir-fry for 3 to 5 minutes longer or until the vegetables are tender and the sauce has thickened.
5. **Serve**

**Nutrition:**

Calories: 361

Fat: 16g

Carbohydrates: 49g

Protein: 8g

Sodium: 95mg

Phosphorus: 267mg

Potassium: 582mg

## 110. Curried Veggies and Rice

**Preparation Time:** 12 minutes
**Cooking Time:** 18 minutes
**Servings:** 4

**Ingredients:**

- 1/4 cup olive oil
- 1 cup long-grain white basmati rice
- 4 garlic cloves, minced
- 2 1/2 teaspoons curry powder
- 1/2 cup sliced shiitake mushrooms
- 1 red bell pepper, chopped
- 1 cup frozen, shelled edamame
- 2 cups low-sodium vegetable broth
- 1/8 teaspoon freshly ground black pepper

**Directions:**

1. Heat the olive oil on medium heat.
2. Add the rice, garlic, curry powder, mushrooms, bell pepper, and edamame; cook, stirring, for 2 minutes.
3. Add the broth and black pepper and bring to a boil.
4. Reduce the heat to low, partially cover the pot, and simmer for 15 to 18 minutes or until the rice is tender. Stir and serve.

**Nutrition:**

Calories: 347

Fat: 16g

Carbohydrates: 44g

Protein: 8g

Sodium: 114mg

Phosphorus: 131mg

Potassium: 334mg

## 111. Spicy Veggie Pancakes

**Preparation Time: 10 minutes**
**Cooking Time: 10 minutes**
**Servings: 4**
**Ingredients:**

- 3 tablespoons olive oil, divided
- 2 small onions, finely chopped
- 1 jalapeño pepper, minced
- 3/4 cup carrot, grated
- 3/4 cup cabbage, finely chopped
- 1 1/2 cups quick-cooking oats
- 3/4 cup of water
- ½ cup whole-wheat flour
- 1 large egg
- 1 large egg white
- 1 teaspoon baking soda
- 1/4 teaspoon cayenne pepper

**Directions:**

1. In a skillet, heat 2 teaspoons oil over medium heat.
2. Sauté the onion, jalapeño, carrot, and cabbage for 4 minutes.
3. While the veggies are cooking, combine the oats, rice, water, flour, egg, egg white, baking soda, and cayenne pepper in a medium bowl until well mixed.
4. Add the cooked vegetables to the mixture and stir to combine.
5. Heat the remaining oil in a large skillet over medium heat.
6. Drop the mixture into the skillet, about 1/3 cup per pancake. Cook for 4 minutes, or until bubbles form on the pancakes' surface and the edges look cooked, then carefully flip them over.
7. Repeat with the remaining mixture and serve.

**Nutrition:**

Calories: 323

Fat: 11g

Carbohydrates: 48g

Protein: 10g

Sodium: 366mg

Potassium: 381mg

Phosphorus: 263mg

## 112. Egg and Veggie Fajitas

**Preparation Time:** 15 minutes

**Cooking Time:** 10 minutes

**Servings:** 4

**Ingredients:**

- 3 large eggs
- 3 egg whites
- 2 teaspoons chili powder
- 1 tablespoon unsalted butter
- 1 onion, chopped
- 2 garlic cloves, minced
- 1 jalapeño pepper, minced
- 1 red bell pepper, chopped
- 1 cup frozen corn, thawed and drained
- 8 (6-inch) corn tortillas

**Directions:**

1. Whisk the eggs, egg whites, and chili powder in a small bowl until well combined. Set aside.
2. Prepare a large skillet and melt the butter on medium heat.
3. Sauté the onion, garlic, jalapeño, bell pepper, and corn until the vegetables are tender, 3 to 4 minutes.
4. Add the beaten egg mixture to the skillet. Cook, occasionally stirring, until the eggs form large curds and are set, 3 to 5 minutes.
5. Meanwhile, soften the corn tortillas as directed on the package.
6. Divide the egg mixture evenly among the softened corn tortillas. Roll the tortillas up and serve.

**Nutrition:**

Calories: 316

Fat 14g

Carbohydrates: 35g

Protein: 14g

Sodium: 167mg

Potassium: 408mg

Phosphorus: 287mg

## 113. Vegetable Biryani

**Preparation Time:** 10 minutes

**Cooking Time:** 15 minutes

Servings: 4

**Ingredients:**
- 2 tablespoons olive oil
- 1 onion, diced
- 4 garlic cloves, minced
- 1 tbsp. peeled and grated fresh ginger root
- 1 cup carrot, grated
- 2 cups chopped cauliflower
- 1 cup thawed frozen baby peas
- 2 teaspoons curry powder
- 1 cup low-sodium vegetable broth
- 3 cups of frozen cooked white rice

**Directions:**
1. Get a skillet and heat the olive oil on medium heat.
2. Add onion, garlic, and ginger root. Sauté, frequently stirring, until tender-crisp, 2 minutes.
3. Add the carrot, cauliflower, peas, and curry powder and cook for 2 minutes longer.
4. Put vegetable broth. Cover the skillet partially, and simmer on low for 6 to 7 minutes or until the vegetables are tender.
5. Meanwhile, heat the rice as directed on the package.
6. Stir the rice into the vegetable mixture and serve.

**Nutrition:**

Calories: 378

Fat 16g

Carbohydrates: 53g

Protein: 8g

Sodium: 113mg

Potassium: 510mg

Phosphorus: 236mg

## 114. Creamy Tuna Salad

**Preparation Time:** 10 minutes

**Cooking Time:** 5 minutes

**Servings:** 4

**Ingredients:**

- 3.5 oz. can tuna, drained and flaked
- 1 1/2 tsp garlic powder
- 1 tbsp. dill, chopped
- 1 tsp curry powder
- 2 tbsp. fresh lemon juice
- 1/2 cup onion, chopped
- 1/2 cup celery, chopped
- 1/4 cup parmesan cheese, grated
- 3/4 cup mayonnaise

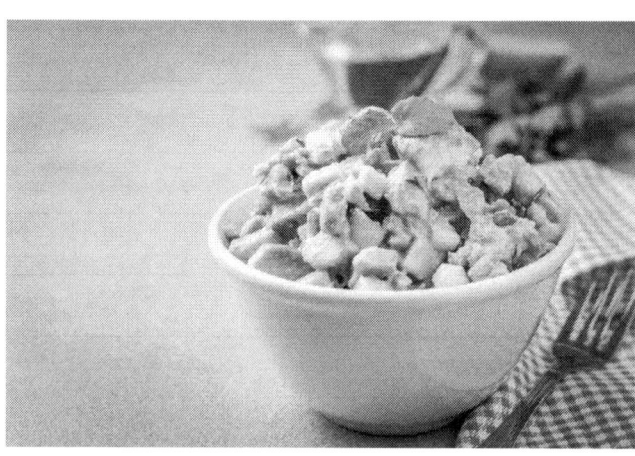

**Directions:**

1. Add all ingredients into the large bowl and mix until well combined.
2. Serve and enjoy.

**Nutrition:** Calories 224 Fat 15.5 g Carbohydrates 14.1 g Sugar 4.2 g Protein 8 g Cholesterol 20 mg Phosphorus: 110mg Potassium: 117mg Sodium: 75mg

## 115. Creamy Mushroom Soup

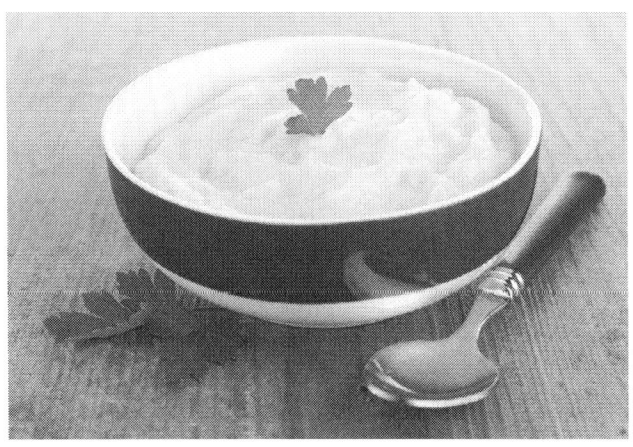

**Preparation Time:** 10 minutes
**Cooking Time:** 15 minutes
**Servings:** 6
**Ingredients:**

- 1 lb. mushrooms, sliced
- 1/2 cup heavy cream
- 4 cups chicken broth
- 1 tbsp. sage, chopped
- 1/4 cup butter
- Pepper
- Salt

**Directions:**

1. Melt butter in a large pot over medium heat.
2. Add sage and saute for 1 minute.
3. Add mushrooms and cook for 3-5 minutes or until lightly browned.
4. Add broth and stir well and simmer for 5 minutes.
5. Puree the soup using an immersion blender until smooth.
6. Add heavy cream and stir well. Season soup with pepper and salt.
7. Serve hot and enjoy.

**Nutrition:** Calories 145 Fat 12.5 g Carbohydrates 3.6 g Sugar 1.8 g Protein 5.9 g Cholesterol 34 mg Phosphorus: 140mg Potassium: 127mg Sodium: 75mg

## 116. Pork Soup

**Preparation Time:** 10 minutes

**Cooking Time:** 4 hours 15 minutes

**Servings:** 8

**Ingredients:**

- 2 lbs. country pork ribs, boneless and cut into 1-inch pieces
- 2 cups cauliflower rice
- 1 1/2 tbsp. fresh oregano, chopped
- 1 cup of water
- 2 cups Red bell peppers, chopped
- 1 cup chicken stock
- 1/2 cup dry white wine
- 1 onion, chopped
- 3 garlic cloves, chopped
- 1 tbsp. olive oil
- Pepper
- Salt

**Directions:**

1. Heat oil in a saucepan over medium heat.
2. Season pork with pepper and salt. Add pork into the saucepan and cook until lightly brown from all the sides.
3. Add onion and garlic and saute for 2 minutes.
4. Add Red bell peppers, water, stock, and white wine and stir well. Bring to boil.
5. Pour saucepan mixture into the slow cooker.
6. Cover and cook on high for 4 hours.
7. Add cauliflower rice and oregano in the last 20 minutes of cooking.
8. Stir well and serve.

**Nutrition:** Calories 263 Fat 15.1 g Carbohydrates 5.8 g Sugar 2.6 g Protein 23.4 g Cholesterol 85 mg Phosphorus: 130mg Potassium: 117mg Sodium: 105mg

## 117. Thai Chicken Soup

**Preparation Time:** 10 minutes
**Cooking Time:** 30 minutes
**Servings:** 6
**Ingredients:**

- 4 chicken breasts, slice into 1/4-inch strips
- 1 tbsp. fresh basil, chopped
- 1 tsp ground ginger
- 1 oz. fresh lime juice
- 1 tbsp. coconut aminos
- 2 tbsp. chili garlic paste
- 1/4 cup fish sauce
- 28 oz. water
- 14 oz. chicken broth
- 14 oz. coconut milk

**Directions:**

1. Add coconut milk, basil, ginger, lime juice, coconut aminos, chili garlic paste, fish sauce, water, and broth into the stockpot. Stir well and bring to boil over medium-high heat.
2. Add chicken and stir well. Turn heat to medium-low and simmer for 30 minutes.
3. Stir well and serve.

**Nutrition:** Calories 357 Fat 23.4 g Carbohydrates 5.5 g Sugar 2.9 g Protein 31.7 g Cholesterol 87 mg Phosphorus: 110mg Potassium: 117mg Sodium: 75mg

## 118. Tasty Pumpkin Soup

**Preparation Time:** 10 minutes
**Cooking Time:** 30 minutes
**Servings:** 6
**Ingredients:**

- 2 cups pumpkin puree
- 1 cup coconut cream
- 4 cups vegetable broth
- 1/2 tsp ground ginger
- 1 tsp curry powder
- 2 shallots, chopped
- 1/2 onion, chopped
- 4 tbsp. butter
- Pepper
- Salt

**Directions:**

1. Melt butter in a saucepan over medium heat.
2. Add shallots and onion and sauté until softened.
3. Add ginger and curry powder and stir well.
4. Add broth, pumpkin puree, and coconut cream and stir well. Simmer for 10 minutes.
5. Puree the soup using an immersion blender until smooth.
6. Season with pepper and salt.
7. Serve and enjoy.

**Nutrition:** Calories 229 Fat 18.4 g Carbohydrates 13 g Sugar 4.9 g Protein 5.6 g Cholesterol 20 mg Phosphorus: 120mg Potassium: 137mg Sodium: 95mg

## 119. Easy Zucchini Soup

**Preparation Time:** 10 minutes

**Cooking Time:** 25 minutes

**Servings:** 4

**Ingredients:**

- 5 zucchinis, sliced
- 8 oz. cream cheese, softened
- 5 cups vegetable stock
- Pepper
- Salt

**Directions:**

1. Add zucchini and stock into the stockpot and bring to boil over high heat.
2. Turn heat to medium and simmer for 20 minutes.
3. Add cream cheese and stir until cheese is melted.
4. Puree soup using an immersion blender until smooth.
5. Season with pepper and salt.
6. Serve and enjoy.

**Nutrition:** Calories 245 Fat 20.3 g Carbohydrates 10.9 g Sugar 5.2 g Protein 7.7 g Cholesterol 62 mg Phosphorus: 110mg Potassium: 117mg Sodium: 75mg

## 120. Quick Tomato Soup

**Preparation Time:** 10 minutes
**Cooking Time:** 5 minutes
**Servings:** 4
**Ingredients:**

- 28 oz. can tomato, diced
- 1 tbsp. balsamic vinegar
- 1 tbsp. dried basil
- 1 tbsp. dried oregano
- 1 tsp garlic, minced
- 2 tbsp. olive oil
- Pepper
- Salt

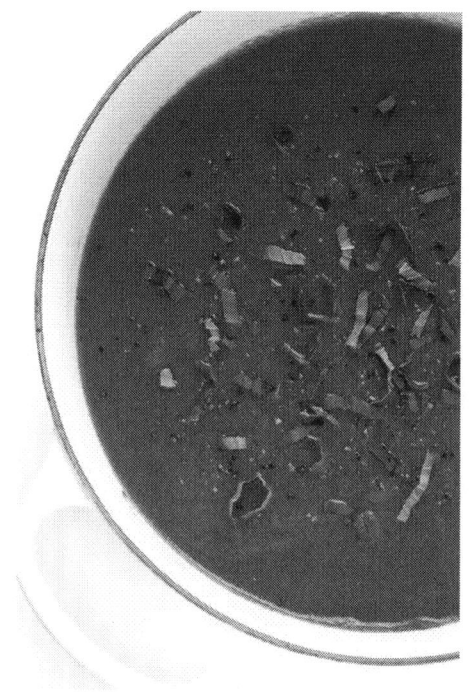

**Directions:**

1. Heat oil in a saucepan over medium heat.
2. Add basil, oregano, and garlic and saute for 30 seconds.
3. Add Red bell peppers, vinegar, pepper, and salt and simmer for 3 minutes.
4. Stir well and serve hot.

**Nutrition:** Calories 108 Fat 7.1 g Carbohydrates 11.2 g Sugar 6.8 g Protein 2 g Cholesterol 0 mg Phosphorus: 130mg Potassium: 127mg Sodium: 75mg

## 121. Spicy Chicken Soup

**Preparation Time:** 10 minutes
**Cooking Time:** 5 minutes
**Servings:** 4
**Ingredients:**

- 2 cups cooked chicken, shredded
- 1/2 cup half and half
- 4 cups chicken broth
- 1/3 cup hot sauce
- 3 tbsp. butter
- 4 oz. cream cheese
- Pepper
- Salt

**Directions:**

1. Add half and half, broth, hot sauce, butter, and cream cheese into the blender and blend until smooth.
2. Pour blended mixture into the saucepan and cook over medium heat until just hot.
3. Add chicken stir well. Season soup with pepper and salt.
4. Serve and enjoy.

**Nutrition:** Calories 361 Fat 25.6 g Carbohydrates 3.3 g Sugar 1.1 g Protein 28.4 g Cholesterol 119 mg Phosphorus: 110mg Potassium: 117mg Sodium: 75mg

## 122. Shredded Pork Soup

**Preparation Time:** 10 minutes

**Cooking Time:** 8 hours

**Servings:** 8

**Ingredients:**

- 1 lb. pork loin
- 8 cups chicken broth
- 2 tsp fresh lime juice
- 1 1/2 tsp garlic powder
- 1 1/2 tsp onion powder
- 1 1/2 tsp chili powder
- 1 1/2 tsp cumin
- 1 jalapeno pepper, minced
- 1 cup onion, chopped
- 3 Red bell peppers, chopped

**Directions:**

1. Add Red bell peppers, jalapeno, and onion into the slow cooker and stir well.
2. Place meat on top of the tomato mixture.
3. Pour remaining ingredients on top of the meat.
4. Cover slow cooker and cook on low for 8 hours.
5. Remove meat from slow cooker and shred using a fork.
6. Return shredded meat to the slow cooker and stir well.
7. Serve and enjoy.

**Nutrition:** Calories 199 Fat 9.6 g Carbohydrates 6.3 g Sugar 3.1 g Protein 21.2 g Cholesterol 45 mg Phosphorus: 140mg Potassium: 127mg Sodium: 95mg

## 123. Creamy Chicken Green lettuce Soup

**Preparation Time:** 10 minutes

**Cooking Time:** 10 minutes

**Servings:** 6

**Ingredients:**

- 3 cups cooked chicken, shredded
- 1/8 tsp nutmeg
- 4 cup chicken broth
- 1/2 cup parmesan cheese, shredded
- 8 oz. cream cheese
- 1/4 cup butter
- 4 cup baby green lettuce, chopped
- 1 tsp garlic, minced
- Pepper
- Salt

**Directions:**

1. Melt butter in a saucepan over medium heat.
2. Add green lettuce and garlic and cook until green lettuce is wilted.
3. Add parmesan cheese and cream cheese and stir until cheese is melted.
4. Add remaining ingredients and stir everything well and cook for 5 minutes.
5. Season soup with pepper and salt.
6. Serve and enjoy.

**Nutrition:** Calories 361 Fat 25.6 g Carbohydrates 2.8 g Sugar 0.6 g Protein 29.5 g Cholesterol 121 mg Phosphorus: 110mg Potassium: 117mg Sodium: 75mg

## 124. Shrimp Paella

**Preparation Time:** 5 minutes
**Cooking Time:** 10 minutes
**Servings:** 2

**Ingredients:**
- 1 cup cooked white rice
- 1 chopped red onion
- 1 tsp. paprika
- 1 chopped garlic clove
- 1 tbsp. olive oil
- 6 oz. frozen cooked shrimp
- 1 deseeded and sliced chili pepper
- 1 tbsp. oregano

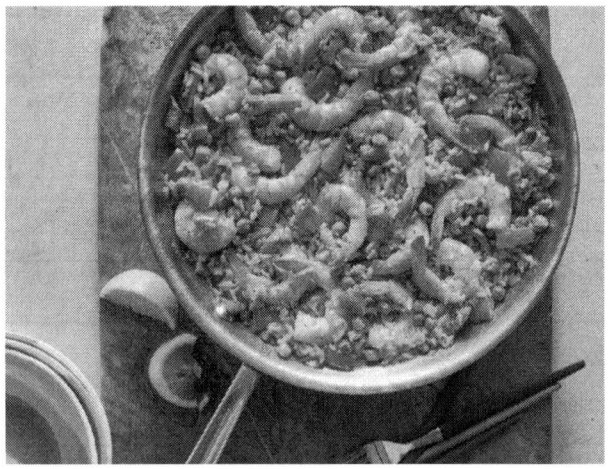

**Directions:**
1. Warm-up olive oil in a large pan on medium-high heat. Add the onion and garlic and sauté for 2-3 minutes until soft. Now add the shrimp and sauté for a further 5 minutes or until hot through.
2. Now add the herbs, spices, chili, and rice with 1/2 cup boiling water. Stir until everything is warm, and the water has been absorbed. Plate up and serve.

**Nutrition:**
Calories 221
Protein 17 g
Carbs 31 g
Fat 8 g
Sodium 235 mg
Potassium 176 mg
Phosphorus 189 mg

## 125. Salmon & Pesto Salad

**Preparation Time:** 5 minutes
**Cooking Time:** 15 minutes
**Servings:** 2
**Ingredients:**

For the pesto:
- 1 minced garlic clove
- ½ cup fresh arugula
- ¼ cup extra virgin olive oil
- ½ cup fresh basil
- 1 tsp black pepper

For the salmon:
- 4 oz. skinless salmon fillet
- 1 tbsp. coconut oil

For the salad:
- ½ juiced lemon
- 2 sliced radishes
- ½ cup iceberg lettuce
- 1 tsp black pepper

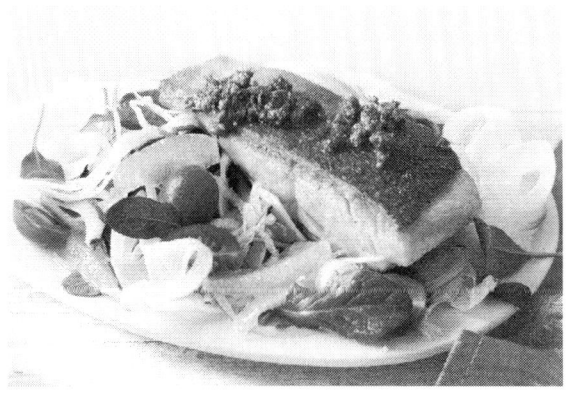

**Directions:**
1. Prepare the pesto by blending all the fixing for the pesto in a food processor or grinding with a pestle and mortar. Set aside.
2. Add a skillet to the stove on medium-high heat and melt the coconut oil. Add the salmon to the pan. Cook for 7-8 minutes and turn over.
3. Cook within 3-4 minutes or until cooked through. Remove fillets from the skillet and allow to rest.
4. Mix the lettuce and the radishes and squeeze over the juice of ½ lemon. Shred the salmon using a fork and mix through the salad. Toss to coat and sprinkle with a little black pepper to serve.

**Nutrition:**

Calories 221

Protein 13 g

Carbs 1 g

Fat 34 g

Sodium 80 mg

Potassium 119 mg

Phosphorus 158 mg

## 126. Baked Fennel & Garlic Sea Bass

**Preparation Time:** 5 minutes
**Cooking Time:** 15 minutes
**Servings:** 2
**Ingredients:**

- 1 lemon
- ½ sliced fennel bulb
- 6 oz. sea bass fillets
- 1 tsp black pepper
- 2 garlic cloves

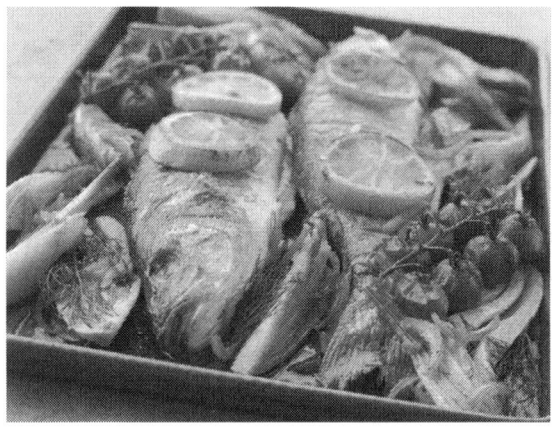

**Directions:**

1. Preheat the oven to 375°F. Sprinkle black pepper over the Sea Bass. Slice the fennel bulb and garlic cloves. Add 1 salmon fillet and half the fennel and garlic to one sheet of baking paper or tin foil.
2. Squeeze in 1/2 lemon juices. Repeat for the other fillet. Fold and add to the oven for 12-15 minutes or until fish is thoroughly cooked through.
3. Meanwhile, add boiling water to your couscous, cover, and allow to steam. Serve with your choice of rice or salad.

**Nutrition:**

Calories 221

Protein 14 g

Carbs 3 g

Fat 2 g

Sodium 119 mg

Potassium 398 mg

Phosphorus 149 mg

## 127. Lemon, Garlic, Cilantro Tuna and Rice

**Preparation Time:** 5 minutes

**Cooking Time:** 0 minutes

**Servings:** 2

**Ingredients:**

- ½ cup arugula
- 1 tbsp. extra virgin olive oil
- 1 cup cooked rice
- 1 tsp black pepper
- ¼ finely diced red onion
- 1 juiced lemon
- 3 oz. canned tuna
- 2 tbsp. Chopped fresh cilantro

**Directions:**

1. Mix the olive oil, pepper, cilantro, and red onion in a bowl. Stir in the tuna, cover, then serve with the cooked rice and arugula!

**Nutrition:**

Calories 221

Protein 11 g

Carbs 26 g

Fat 7 g

Sodium 143 mg

Potassium 197 mg

Phosphorus 182 mg

## 128. Cod & Green Bean Risotto

**Preparation Time:** 4 minutes
**Cooking Time:** 40 minutes
**Servings:** 2

**Ingredients:**

- ½ cup arugula
- 1 finely diced white onion
- 4 oz. cod fillet
- 1 cup white rice
- 2 lemon wedges
- 1 cup boiling water
- ¼ tsp. black pepper
- 1 cup low-sodium chicken broth
- 1 tbsp. extra virgin olive oil
- ½ cup green beans

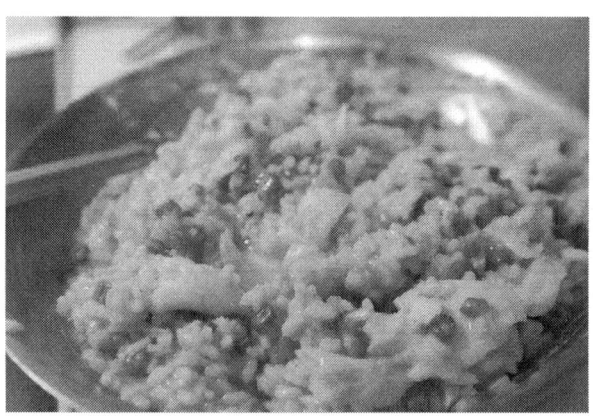

**Directions:**

1. Warm-up oil in a large pan on medium heat. Sauté the chopped onion for 5 minutes until soft before adding in the rice and stirring for 1-2 minutes.
2. Combine the broth with boiling water. Add half of the liquid to the pan and stir. Slowly add the rest of the liquid while continuously stirring for up to 20-30 minutes.
3. Stir in the green beans to the risotto. Place the fish on top of the rice, cover, and steam for 10 minutes.
4. Use your fork to break up the fish fillets and stir into the rice. Sprinkle with freshly ground pepper to serve and a squeeze of fresh lemon. Serve with the lemon wedges and the arugula.

**Nutrition:**

Calories 221

Protein 12 g

Carbs 29 g

Fat 8 g

Sodium 398 mg

Potassium 347 mg

Phosphorus 241 mg

## 129. Sardine Fish Cakes

**Preparation Time:** 10 minutes

**Cooking Time:** 10 minutes

**Servings:** 4

**Ingredients:**

- 11 oz. sardines, canned, drained
- 1/3 cup shallot, chopped
- 1 teaspoon chili flakes
- ½ teaspoon salt
- 2 tablespoon wheat flour, whole grain
- 1 egg, beaten
- 1 tablespoon chives, chopped
- 1 teaspoon olive oil
- 1 teaspoon butter

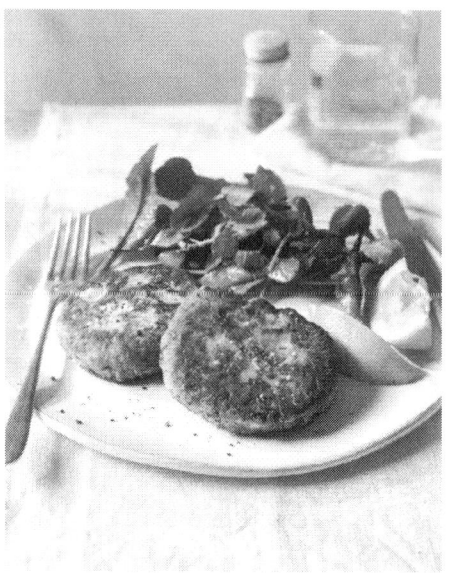

**Directions:**

1. Put the butter in your skillet and dissolve it. Add shallot and cook it until translucent. After this, transfer the shallot to the mixing bowl.
2. Add sardines, chili flakes, salt, flour, egg, chives, and mix up until smooth with the fork's help. Make the medium size cakes and place them in the skillet. Add olive oil.
3. Roast the fish cakes for 3 minutes from each side over medium heat. Dry the cooked fish cakes with a paper towel if needed and transfer to the serving plates.

**Nutrition:**

Calories 221

Fat 12.2g

Fiber 0.1g

Carbs 5.4g

Protein 21.3 g

Phosphorus 188.7 mg

Potassium 160.3 mg

Sodium 452.6 mg

## 130. 4-Ingredients Salmon Fillet

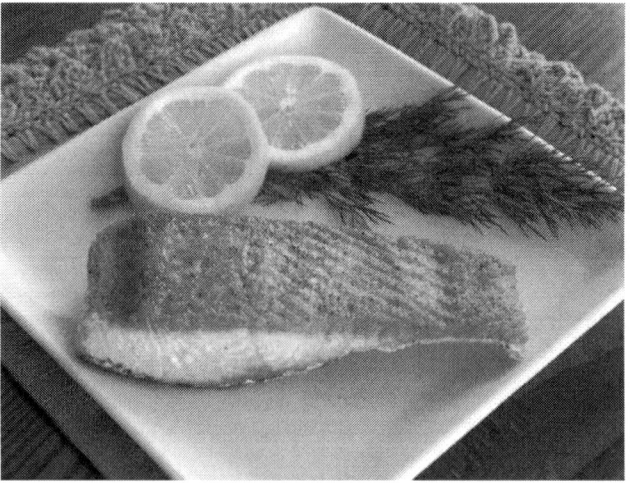

**Preparation Time:** 5 minutes

**Cooking Time:** 25 minutes

Servings: 1

**Ingredients:**

- 4 oz. salmon fillet
- ½ teaspoon salt
- 1 teaspoon sesame oil
- ½ teaspoon sage

**Directions:**

1. Rub the fillet with salt and sage. Put the fish in the tray, then sprinkle it with sesame oil. Cook the fish for 25 minutes at 365F. Flip the fish carefully onto another side after 12 minutes of cooking. Serve.

**Nutrition:**

Calories 191

Fat 11.6g

Fiber 0.1g

Carbs 0.2g

Protein 22g

Sodium 70.5 mg

Phosphorus 472 mg

Potassium 636.3 mg

## 131. Spanish Cod in Sauce

**Preparation Time:** 10 minutes

**Cooking Time:** 5 1/2 hours

**Servings:** 2

**Ingredients:**

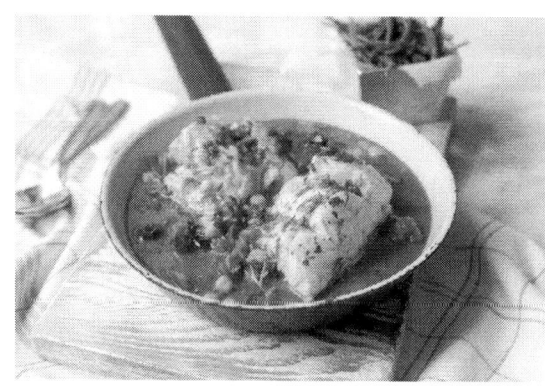

- 1 teaspoon tomato paste
- 1 teaspoon garlic, diced
- 1 white onion, sliced
- 1 jalapeno pepper, chopped
- 1/3 cup chicken stock
- 7 oz. Spanish cod fillet
- 1 teaspoon paprika
- 1 teaspoon salt

**Directions:**

1. Pour chicken stock into the saucepan. Add tomato paste and mix up the liquid until homogenous. Add garlic, onion, jalapeno pepper, paprika, and salt.
2. Bring the liquid to boil and then simmer it. Chop the cod fillet and add it to the tomato liquid. Simmer the fish for 10 minutes over low heat. Serve the fish in the bowls with tomato sauce.

**Nutrition:**

Calories 113

Fat 1.2g

Fiber 1.9g

Carbs 7.2g

Protein 18.9g

Potassium 659 mg

Sodium 597 mg

Phosphorus 18 mg

## 132. Salmon Baked in Foil with Fresh Thyme

**Preparation Time:** 10 minutes

**Cooking Time:** 30 minutes

**Servings:** 4

**Ingredients:**

- 4 fresh thyme sprigs
- 4 garlic cloves, peeled, roughly chopped
- 16 oz. salmon fillets (4 oz. each fillet)
- ½ teaspoon salt
- ½ teaspoon ground black pepper
- 4 tablespoons cream
- 4 teaspoons butter
- ¼ teaspoon cumin seeds

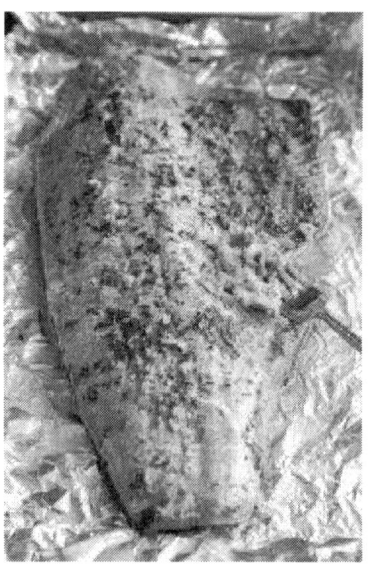

**Directions:**

1. Line the baking tray with foil. Sprinkle the fish fillets with salt, ground black pepper, cumin seeds, and arrange them in the tray with oil.
2. Add thyme sprig on the top of every fillet. Then add cream, butter, and garlic. Bake the fish for 30 minutes at 345F. Serve.

**Nutrition:**

Calories 198

Fat 11.6g

Carbs 1.8g

Protein 22.4g

Phosphorus 425 mg

Potassium 660.9 mg

Sodium 366 mg

## 133. Poached Halibut in Orange Sauce

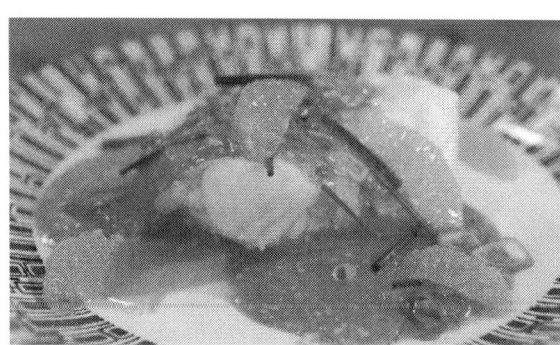

**Preparation Time:** 10 minutes
**Cooking Time:** 10 minutes
**Servings:** 4
**Ingredients:**
- 1-pound halibut
- 1/3 cup butter
- 1 rosemary sprig
- ½ teaspoon ground black pepper
- 1 teaspoon salt
- 1 teaspoon honey
- ¼ cup of orange juice
- 1 teaspoon cornstarch

**Directions:**
1. Put butter in the saucepan and melt it. Add rosemary sprig. Sprinkle the halibut with salt and ground black pepper. Put the fish in the boiling butter and poach it for 4 minutes.
2. Meanwhile, pour orange juice into the skillet. Add honey and bring the liquid to boil. Add cornstarch and whisk until the liquid starts to be thick. Then remove it from the heat.
3. Transfer the poached halibut to the plate and cut it on 4. Place every fish serving in the serving plate and top with orange sauce.

**Nutrition:**
Calories 349
Fat 29.3g
Fiber 0.1g
Carbs 3.2g
Protein 17.8g
Phosphorus 154 mg
Potassium 388.6 mg
Sodium 29.3 mg

# CHAPTER 8:

# Snack Recipes

## 134. Veggie Snack

**Preparation Time: 5 minutes**
**Cooking Time: 10 minutes**
**Servings: 1**
**Ingredients:**

- 1 large yellow pepper
- 5 carrots
- 5 stalks celery

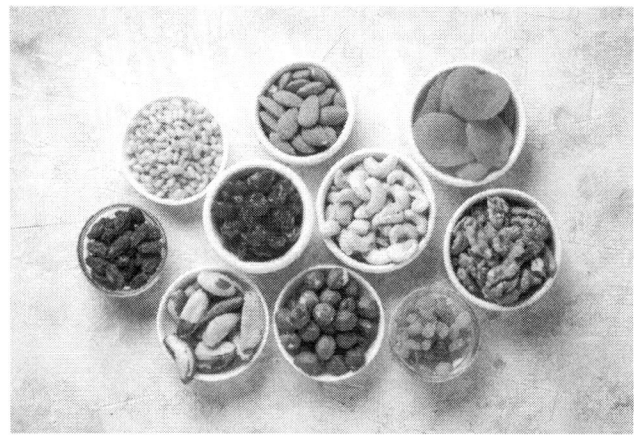

**Directions:**

1. Clean the carrots and rinse under running water.
2. Rinse celery and yellow pepper. Remove seeds of pepper and chop the veggies into small sticks.
3. Put in a bowl and serve.

**Nutrition:**

Calories: 189

Fat: 0.5 g

Carbs: 44.3 g

Protein: 5 g

Sodium: 282 mg

Potassium: 0mg

Phosphorus: 0mg

## 135. Healthy Spiced Nuts

**Preparation Time:** 10 minutes

**Cooking Time:** 10 minutes

**Servings:** 4

**Ingredients:**

- 1 tbsp. extra virgin olive oil
- ¼ cup walnuts
- ¼ cup pecans
- ¼ cup almonds
- ½ tsp. sea salt
- ½ tsp. cumin
- ½ tsp. pepper
- 1 tsp. chili powder

**Directions:**

1. Put the skillet on medium heat and toast the nuts until lightly browned.
2. Prepare the spice mixture and add black pepper, cumin, chili, and salt.
3. Put extra virgin olive oil and sprinkle with spice mixture to the toasted nuts before serving.

**Nutrition:**

Calories: 88

Fat: 8g

Carbs: 4g

Protein: 2.5g

Sodium: 51mg

Potassium: 88mg

Phosphorus: 6.3mg

## 136. Roasted Asparagus

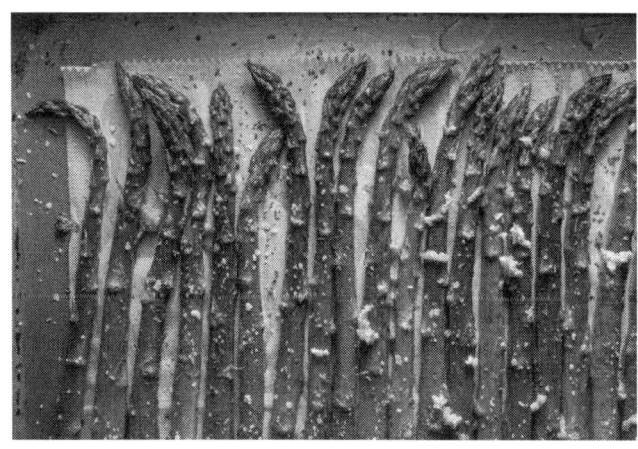

**Preparation Time:** 5 minutes
**Cooking Time:** 10 minutes
**Servings:** 4
**Ingredients:**

- 1 tbsp. extra virgin olive oil
- 1-pound fresh asparagus
- 1 medium lemon, zested
- 1/2 tsp. freshly grated nutmeg
- 1/2 tsp. kosher salt
- ½ tsp. black pepper

**Directions:**

1. Preheat your oven to 500 degrees F.
2. Put asparagus on an aluminum foil and add extra virgin olive oil.
3. Prepare asparagus in a single layer and fold the edges of the foil.
4. Cook in the oven for 5 minutes. Continue roasting until browned.
5. Add the roasted asparagus with nutmeg, salt, zest, and pepper before serving.

**Nutrition:**

Calories: 55
Fat: 3.8 g
Carbs: 4.7 g
Protein: 2.5 g
Sodium: 98mg
Potassium: 172mg
Phosphorus: 35mg

## 137. Low-Fat Mango Salsa

**Preparation Time:** 10 minutes

**Cooking Time:** 10 minutes

**Servings:** 4

**Ingredients:**

- 1 cup cucumber, chopped
- 2 cups mango, diced
- ½ cup cilantro, minced
- 2 tablespoons fresh lime juice
- 1 tablespoon scallions, minced
- ¼ teaspoon chipotle powder
- ¼ teaspoon sea salt

**Directions**

1. Mix the ingredients in a bowl and serve or refrigerate.

**Nutrition:**

Calories: 155

Fat: 0.6 g

Carbs: 38.2 g

Protein: 1.4 g

Sodium: 3.2 mg

Potassium: 221mg

Phosphorus: 27mg

## 138. Vinegar & Salt Kale

**Preparation Time:** 10 minutes
**Cooking Time:** 12 minutes
**Servings:** 2
**Ingredients:**

- 1 head kale, chopped
- 1 teaspoon extra virgin olive oil
- 1 tablespoon apple cider vinegar
- ½ teaspoon of sea salt

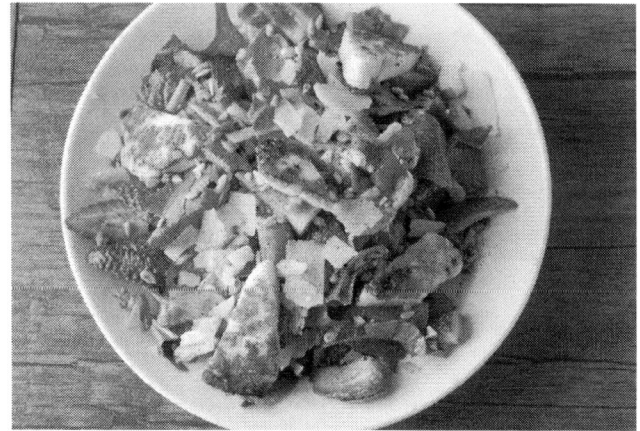

**Directions:**

2. Prepare kale in a bowl and put vinegar and extra virgin olive oil.
3. Sprinkle with salt and massage the ingredients with hands.
4. Spread the kale out onto two paper-lined baking sheets and bake at 375°F for about 12 minutes or until crispy.
5. Let cool for about 10 minutes before serving.

**Nutrition:**

Calories: 152

Fat: 8.2 g

Carbs: 15.2 g

Protein: 4 g

Sodium: 170mg

Potassium: 304mg

Phosphorus: 37mg

## 139. Carrot and Parsnips French Fries

**Preparation Time: 15 minutes**

**Cooking Time: 20 minutes**

Servings: 2

**Ingredients:**

- 6 large carrots
- 6 large parsnips
- 2 tablespoons extra virgin olive oil
- ½ teaspoon of sea salt

**Directions:**

1. Chop the carrots and parsnips into 2-inch slices and then cut each into thin sticks.
2. Toss together the carrots and parsnip sticks with extra virgin olive oil and salt in a bowl and spread into a baking sheet lined with parchment paper.
3. Bake the sticks at 425° for about 20 minutes or until browned.

**Nutrition:**

Calories: 179

Fat: 4g

Carbs: 14g

Protein: 11g

Sodium: 27.3mg

Potassium: 625mg

Phosphorus: 116mg

## 140. Apple & Strawberry Snack

**Preparation Time: 5 minutes**

**Cooking Time: 2 minutes**

**Servings: 1**

**Ingredients:**

- ½ apple, cored and sliced
- 2-3 strawberries
- dash of ground cinnamon
- 2-3 drops stevia 2-3 drops

**Directions:**

1. In a bowl, mix strawberries and apples and sprinkle with stevia and cinnamon.
2. Microwave for about 1-2 minutes. Serve warm.

**Nutrition:**

Calories: 145

Fat: 0.8 g

Carbs: 34.2 g

Protein: 1.6 g

Sodium: 20 mg

Potassium: 0mg

Phosphorus: 0mg

## 141. Candied Macadamia Nuts

**Preparation Time: 5 minutes**
**Cooking Time: 15 minutes**
Servings: 2

**Ingredients:**

- 2 cups macadamia nuts
- 1 tablespoon extra-virgin olive oil
- 2 tablespoons honey

**Directions:**

1. Toss ingredients in bowl and spread into a baking dish.
2. Bake for 15 minutes at 350°F.
3. Let cool before serving.

**Nutrition:**

Calories: 200

Fat: 18 g

Carbs: 10g

Protein: 1g

Sodium: 5 mg

Potassium: 55mg

Phosphorus: 10mg

## 142. Cinnamon Apple Fries

**Preparation Time:** 5 minutes
**Cooking Time:** 15 minutes
**Servings:** 1
**Ingredients:**

- 1 apple, sliced thinly
- Dash of cinnamon
- Stevia

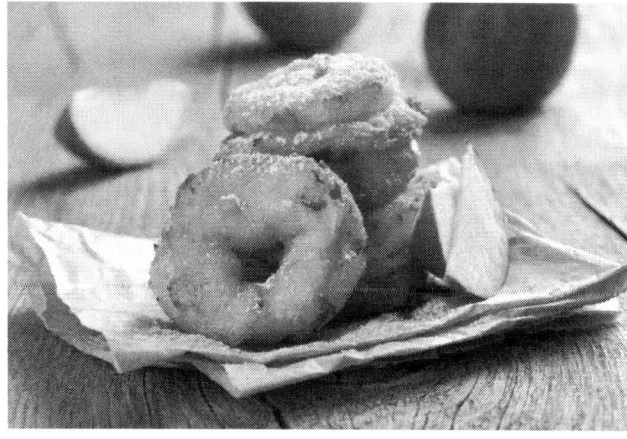

**Directions:**

1. Coat apple slices with cinnamon and stevia.
2. Bake for 15 minutes or until tender and crispy at 325 degrees F.

**Nutrition:**

Calories: 146

Fat: 0.7 g

Carbs: 36.4 g

Protein: 1.6 g

Sodium: 10 mg

Potassium: 100mg

Phosphorus: 0mg

## 143. Lemon Pops

**Preparation Time: 5 minutes**

**Cooking Time: 5 minutes**

**Servings: 1**

**Ingredients:**

- 4 tablespoons fresh lemon juice
- Powdered stevia

**Directions:**

1. Mix orange or lemon juice and stevia and pour into molds.
2. Freeze until firm.

**Nutrition:**

Calories: 46

Fat: 0.2g

Carbs: 16g

Protein: 0.9g

Sodium: 3.7mg

Potassium: 104mg

Phosphorus: 11mg

## 144. Easy No-Bake Coconut Cookies

**Preparation Time:** 5 minutes

**Cooking Time:** 10 minutes

**Servings:** 20

**Ingredients:**

- 3 cups finely shredded coconut flakes
- 1 cup melted coconut oil
- 1 teaspoon liquid stevia

**Directions:**

1. Prepare all ingredients in a large bowl; stir until well blended.
2. Form the mixture into small balls and arrange them on a paper-lined baking tray.
3. Press each cookie down with a fork and refrigerate until firm. Enjoy!

**Nutrition:**

Calories: 99

Fat: 10 g

Carbs: 2 g

Protein: 3 g

Sodium: 7 mg

Potassium: 105mg

Phosphorus: 11mg

## 145. Roasted Chili-Vinegar Peanuts

**Preparation Time:** 5 minutes

**Cooking Time:** 10 minutes

**Servings:** 4

**Ingredients:**

- 1 tablespoon coconut oil
- 2 cups raw peanuts, unsalted
- 2 teaspoon sea salt
- 2 tablespoon apple cider vinegar
- 1 teaspoon chili powder
- 1 teaspoon fresh lime zest

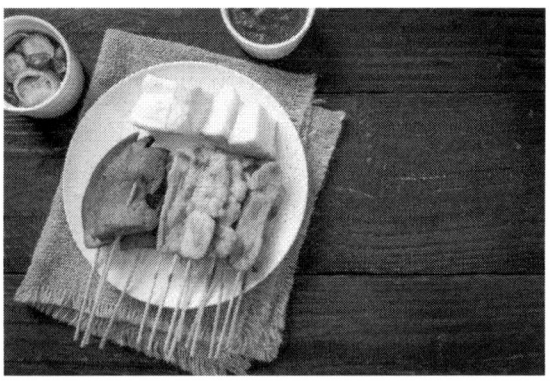

**Directions:**

1. Preheat oven to 350°F.
2. In a large bowl, toss together coconut oil, peanuts, and salt until well coated.
3. Transfer to a rimmed baking sheet and roast in the oven for about 15 minutes or until fragrant.
4. Transfer the roasted peanuts to a bowl and add vinegar, chili powder, and lime zest.
5. Toss to coat well and serve.

**Nutrition:**

Calories: 447

Fat: 39.5g

Carbs: 12.3 g

Protein: 18.9 g

Sodium: 160 mg

Potassium: 200mg

Phosphorus: 0mg

## 146. Popcorn with Sugar and Spice

**Preparation Time: 10 minutes**

**Cooking Time: 10 minutes**

Servings: 2

Ingredients:
- 8 cups hot popcorn
- 2 tablespoons unsalted butter
- 2 tablespoons sugar
- 1/2 teaspoon cinnamon
- 1/4 teaspoon nutmeg

**Directions:**
1. Popping the corn; put aside.
2. Heat the butter, sugar, cinnamon, and nutmeg in the microwave or saucepan over a range fire until the butter is melted, and the sugar dissolved.
3. Sprinkle the corn with the spicy butter, mix well.
4. Serve immediately for optimal flavor.

**Nutrition:**

Calories: 120

Fat: 7g

Carbs: 12g

Protein: 2g

Sodium: 2mg

Potassium: 56mg

Phosphorus: 60mg

## 147. Eggplant and Chickpea Bites

**Preparation Time:** 15 minutes

**Cooking Time:** 50 minutes

**Servings:** 6

**Ingredients:**

- 3 large aubergine cut in half (make a few cuts in the flesh with a knife)
- 2 large cloves garlic, peeled and deglazed
- 2 tbsp. coriander powder
- 2 tbsp. cumin seeds
- 400 g canned chickpeas, rinsed and drained
- 2 Tbsp. chickpea flour
- Zest and juice of 1/2 lemon
- 1/2 lemon quartered for serving
- 3 tbsp. tablespoon of polenta

**Directions:**

1. Heat the oven to 200°C. Spray the eggplant halves generously with oil and place them on the meat side up on a baking sheet.
2. Sprinkle with coriander and cumin seeds, and then place the cloves of garlic on the plate.
3. Season and roast for 40 minutes until the flesh of eggplant is completely tender. Reserve and let cool a little.
4. Scrape the flesh of the eggplant in a bowl with a spatula and throw the skins in the compost. Thoroughly scrape and make sure to incorporate spices and crushed roasted garlic.
5. Add chickpeas, chickpea flour, zest, and lemon juice. Crush roughly and mix well.
6. Check to season. Do not worry if the mixture seems a bit soft - it will firm up in the fridge.
7. Form about twenty pellets and place them on a baking sheet covered with parchment paper. Refrigerate for at least 30 minutes.
8. Preheat oven to 180°C. Remove the meatballs from the fridge and coat them by rolling them in the polenta.
9. Place them back on the baking sheet and spray a little oil on each. Roast for 20 minutes until golden and crisp.
10. Serve with lemon wedges. You can also serve these dumplings with a spicy yogurt dip.

**Nutrition:**

Calories: 72 Fat: 1g Carbs: 18g Protein: 3g Sodium: 63mg Potassium: 162mg Phosphorus: 36mg

## 148. Baba Ghanouj

**Preparation Time:** 10 minutes
**Cooking Time:** 1 hour and 20 minutes
**Servings:** 1
**Ingredients:**

- 1 large aubergine, cut in half lengthwise
- 1 head of garlic, unpeeled
- 30 ml (2 tablespoons) of olive oil
- Lemon juice to taste

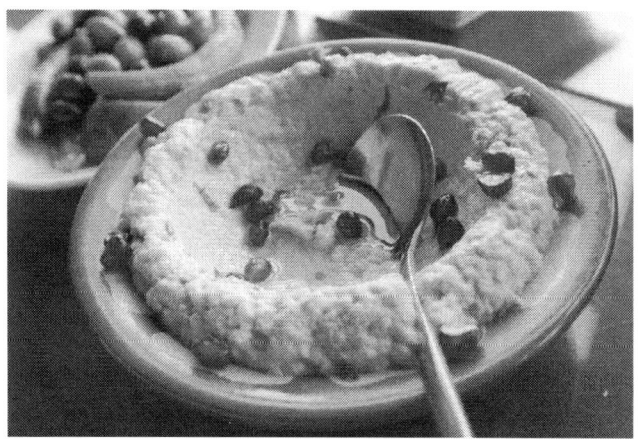

**Directions:**

1. Preheat the oven to 350 degrees F.
2. Place the eggplant on the plate, skin side up. Roast until the meat is very tender and detaches easily from the skin, about 1 hour depending on the eggplant's size. Let cool.
3. Meanwhile, cut the tip of the garlic cloves. Put garlic cloves in a square aluminum foil. Fold the edges of the sheet and fold together to form a tightly wrapped foil.
4. Roast with the eggplant until tender, about 20 minutes. Let cool. Purée the pods with a garlic press.
5. With a spoon, scoop out the eggplant's flesh and place it in the bowl of a food processor. Add the garlic puree, the oil, and the lemon juice. Stir until purée is smooth and pepper.
6. Serve with mini pita bread.

**Nutrition:**

Calories: 110
Fat: 12g
Carbs: 5g
Protein: 1g
Sodium: 180mg
Potassium: 207mg
Phosphorus: 81mg

## 149. Baked Pita Fries

**Preparation Time:** 5 minutes
**Cooking Time:** 15 minutes
**Servings:** 6

**Ingredients:**
- 3 pita loaves (6 inches)
- 3 tablespoons olive oil
- Chili powder

**Directions:**
1. Separate each bread in half with scissors to obtain 6 round pieces.
2. Cut each piece into eight points. Brush each with olive oil and sprinkle with chili powder.
3. Bake at 350 degrees F for about 15 minutes until crisp.

**Nutrition:**
Calories: 120
Fat: 2.5g
Carbs: 22g
Protein: 3g
Sodium: 70mg
Potassium: 0mg
Phosphorus: 0mg

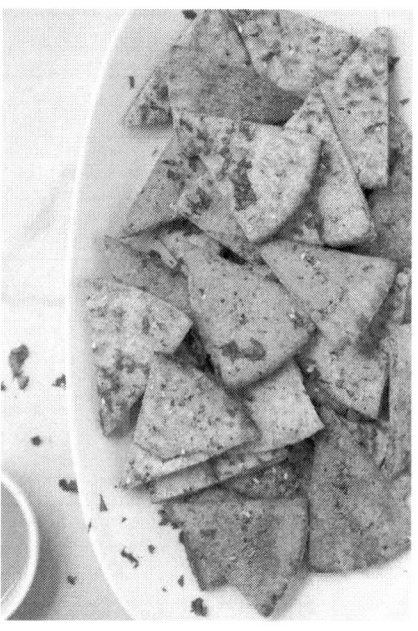

## 150. Herbal Cream Cheese Tartines

**Preparation Time: 15 minutes**

**Cooking Time: 15 minutes**

Servings: 2

Ingredients:
- 1 clove garlic, halved
- 1 cup cream cheese spread
- ¼ cup chopped herbs such as chives, dill, parsley, tarragon, or thyme
- 2 tbsp. minced French shallot or onion
- ½ tsp. black pepper
- 2 tbsp. tablespoons water

Directions:
1. In a medium-sized bowl, combine the cream cheese, herbs, shallot, pepper, and water with a hand blender.
2. Serve the cream cheese with the rusks.

**Nutrition:**

Calories: 476

Fat: 9g

Carbs: 75g

Protein: 23g

Sodium: 885mg

Potassium: 312mg

Phosphorus: 165mg

## 151. Mixes of Snacks

**Preparation Time:** 15 minutes

**Cooking Time:** 1 hour

**Servings:** 1

**Ingredients:**

- 6 c. margarine
- 2 tbsp. Worcestershire sauce
- 1 ½ tbsp. spice salt
- ¾ c. garlic powder
- ½ tsp. onion powder
- 3 cups Cheerios
- 3 cups corn flakes
- 1 cup pretzel
- 1 cup broken bagel chip into 1-inch pieces

**Directions:**

1. Preheat the oven to 250F (120C)
2. Melt the margarine in a large roasting pan. Stir in the seasoning. Gradually add the ingredients remaining by mixing so that the coating is uniform.
3. Cook 1 hour, stirring every 15 minutes.
4. Spread on paper towels to let cool. Store in a tightly closed container.

**Nutrition:**

Calories: 150

Fat: 6g

Carbs: 20g

Protein: 3g

Sodium: 300mg

Potassium: 93mg

Phosphorus: 70mg

## 152. Spicy Crab Dip

**Preparation Time:** 10 minutes

**Cooking Time:** 20 minutes

Servings: 1

**Ingredients:**

- 1 can of 8 oz. softened cream cheese
- 1 tbsp. finely chopped onions
- 1 tbsp. lemon juice
- 2 tbsp. Worcestershire sauce
- 1/8 tsp. black pepper Cayenne pepper to taste
- 2 tbsp. to s. of milk or non-fortified rice drink
- 1 can of 6 oz. of crabmeat

**Directions:**

1. Preheat the oven to 375 degrees F.
2. Pour the cheese cream into a bowl. Add the onions, lemon juice, Worcestershire sauce, black pepper, and cayenne pepper. Mix well. Stir in the milk/rice drink.
3. Add the crabmeat and mix until you obtain a homogeneous mixture.
4. Pour the mixture into a baking dish. Cook without covering for 15 minutes or until bubbles appear. Serve hot with triangle cut pita bread.
5. Microwave until bubbles appear, about 4 minutes, stirring every 1 to 2 minutes.

**Nutrition:**

Calories: 42

Fat: 0.5g

Carbs: 2g

Protein: 7g

Sodium: 167mg

Potassium: 130mg

Phosphorus: 139mg

## 153. Baked Apples with Cherries and Walnuts

**Preparation Time:** 10 minutes

**Cooking Time:** 35 to 40 minutes

**Servings:** 6

**Ingredients:**

- 1/3 cup dried cherries, coarsely chopped
- 3 tablespoons chopped walnuts
- 1 tablespoon ground flaxseed meal
- 1 tablespoon firmly packed brown sugar
- 1 teaspoon ground cinnamon
- 1/8 teaspoon nutmeg
- 6 Golden Delicious apples, about 2 pounds total weight, washed and unpeeled
- 1/2 cup 100 percent apple juice
- 1/4 cup water
- 2 tablespoons dark honey
- 2 teaspoons extra-virgin olive oil

**Directions:**

1. Preheat the oven to 350°F.
2. In a small bowl, toss together the cherries, walnuts, flaxseed meal, brown sugar, cinnamon, and nutmeg until all the ingredients are evenly distributed. Set aside.
3. Working from the stem end, core each apple, stopping ¾ of an inch from the bottom.
4. Gently press the cherries into each apple cavity. Arrange the apples upright in a heavy ovenproof skillet or baking dish just large enough to hold them.
5. Pour the apple juice and water into the pan.
6. Drizzle the honey and oil evenly over the apples, and cover the pan snugly with aluminum foil. Bake until the apples are tender when pierced with a knife, 35 to 40 minutes.
7. Transfer the apples to individual plates and drizzle with the pan juices. Serve warm.

**NUTRITION:** Calories: 162; Total Fat 5g; Saturated Fat: 1g; Cholesterol: 0mg; Sodium: 4mg; Potassium: 148mg; Total Carbohydrate: 30g; Fiber: 4g; Protein: 1g

## 154. Easy Peach Crumble

**Preparation Time:** 10 minutes

**Cooking Time:** 30 minutes

**Servings:** 8

**Ingredients:**
- 8 ripe peaches, peeled, pitted and sliced
- 3 tablespoons freshly squeezed lemon juice
- 1/2 teaspoon ground cinnamon
- 1/4 teaspoon ground nutmeg
- 1/2 cup oat flour
- 1/4 cup packed dark brown sugar
- 2 tablespoons margarine, cut into thin slices
- 1/4 cup quick-cooking oats

**Directions:**
1. Preheat the oven to 375°F. Lightly coat a 9-inch pie pan with cooking spray. Arrange peach slices in the prepared pie plate and sprinkle with the lemon juice, cinnamon, and nutmeg.
2. In a small bowl, whisk together the flour and brown sugar. With your fingers, crumble the margarine into the flour-sugar mixture. Add the uncooked oats and stir to mix. Sprinkle the flour mixture over the peaches.
3. Bake until the peaches are soft and the topping is browned, about 30 minutes.
4. Cut into 8 even slices and serve warm.

**NUTRITION:** Calories: 130; Total Fat 4g; Saturated Fat: 0g; Cholesterol: 0mg; Sodium: 42mg; Potassium: 255mg; Total Carbohydrate: 28g; Fiber: 3g; Protein: 2g

# CHAPTER 9:

# 40 Recipes for those Who Have Dialysis:

# Breakfast

## 155. Breakfast Salad from Grains and Fruits

**Preparation Time:** 5 minutes

**Cooking Time:** 15 minutes

Servings: 6

Ingredients:

- 1 8-oz low fat vanilla yogurt
- 1 orange
- 1 Red delicious apple
- 1 Granny Smith apple
- ¾ cup bulgur
- ¼ teaspoon salt
- 3 cups water

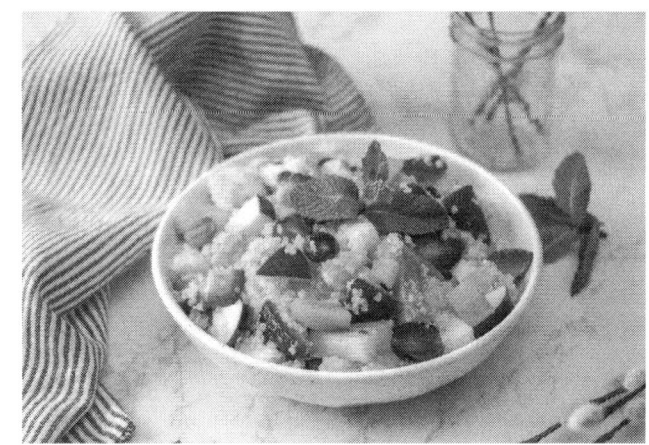

**Direction:**

1. On high fire, place a large pot and bring water to a boil.
2. Add bulgur and rice. Lower fire to a simmer and cooks for ten minutes while covered.
3. Turn off fire, set aside for 2 minutes while covered.
4. In baking sheet, transfer and evenly spread grains to cool.
5. Meanwhile, peel oranges and cut into sections. Chop and core apples.
6. Once grains are cool, transfer to a large serving bowl along with fruits.
7. Add yogurt and mix well to coat.
8. Serve and enjoy.

**Nutrition:**

Calories: 187; Carbs: g; Protein: g;

Fats: g; Phosphorus: mg; Potassium: mg; Sodium: 117mg

## 156. French toast with Applesauce

**Preparation Time:** 5 minutes

**Cooking Time:** 15 minutes

**Servings:** 6

**Ingredients:**
- ¼ cup unsweetened applesauce
- ½ cup milk
- 1 teaspoon ground cinnamon
- 2 eggs
- 2 tablespoon white sugar

**Directions:**
1. Mix well applesauce, sugar, cinnamon, milk and eggs in a mixing bowl.
2. Soak the bread, one by one into applesauce mixture until wet.
3. On medium fire, heat a nonstick skillet greased with cooking spray.
4. Add soaked bread one at a time and cook for 2-3 minutes per side or until lightly browned.
5. Serve and enjoy.

**Nutrition:**

Calories: 57;

Carbs: 6g;

Protein: 4g;

Fats: 4g;

Phosphorus: 69mg;

Potassium: 88mg;

Sodium: 43mg

## 157. Bagels Made Healthy

**Preparation Time:** 5 minutes

**Cooking Time:** 25 minutes

Servings: 8

Ingredients:
- 2 teaspoon yeast
- 1 ½ tablespoon olive oil
- 1 ¼ cups bread flour
- 2 cups whole wheat flour
- 1 tablespoon vinegar
- 2 tablespoon honey
- 1 ½ cups warm water

Directions:
1. In a bread machine, mix all ingredients, and then process on dough cycle.
2. Once done or end of cycle, create 8 pieces shaped like a flattened ball.
3. In the centre of each ball, make a hole using your thumb then create a donut shape.
4. In a greased baking sheet, place donut-shaped dough then covers and let it rise about ½ hour.
5. Prepare about 2 inches of water to boil in a large pan.
6. In a boiling water, drop one at a time the bagels and boil for 1 minute, then turn them once.
7. Remove them and return them to baking sheet and bake at 350oF (175oC) for about 20 to 25 minutes until golden brown.

Nutrition:

Calories: 221;

Carbs: 42g;

Protein: 7g;

Fats: g;

Phosphorus: 130mg;

Potassium: 166mg;

Sodium: 47mg

## 158. Cornbread with Southern Twist

**Preparation Time:** 15 minutes

**Cooking Time:** 60 minutes

**Servings:** 8

**Ingredients:**

- 2 tablespoons shortening
- 1 ¼ cups skim milk
- ¼ cup egg substitute
- 4 tablespoons sodium free baking powder
- ½ cup flour
- 1 ½ cups cornmeal

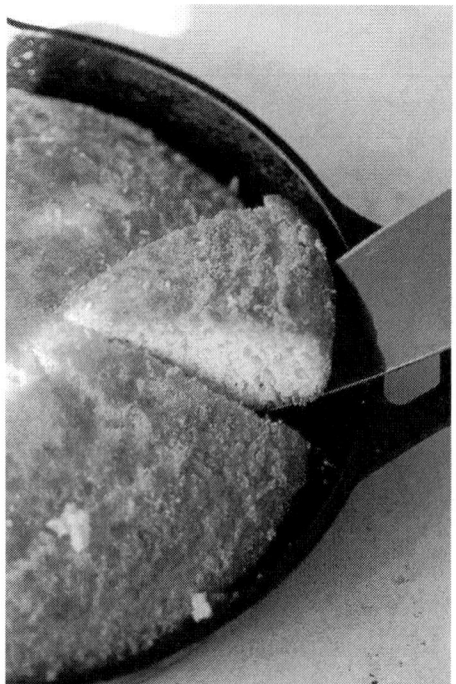

**Directions:**

1. Prepare 8 x 8-inch baking dish or a black iron skillet then add shortening.
2. Put the baking dish or skillet inside the oven on 425oF, once the shortening has melted that means the pan is hot already.
3. In a bowl, add milk and egg then mix well.
4. Take out the skillet and add the melted shortening into the batter and stir well.
5. Pour all mixed ingredients into skillet.
6. For 15 to 20 minutes, cook in the oven until golden brown.

**Nutrition:**

Calories: 166;

Carbs: 35g;

Protein: 5g;

Fats: 1g;

Phosphorus: 79mg;

Potassium: 122mg;

Sodium: 34mg

## 159. Grandma's Pancake Special

**Preparation Time:** 5 minutes

**Cooking Time:** 15 minutes

Servings: 3

Ingredients:

- 1 tablespoon oil
- 1 cup milk
- 1 egg
- 2 teaspoons sodium free baking powder
- 2 tablespoons sugar
- 1 ¼ cups flour

Directions:

1. Mix together all the dry ingredients such as the flour, sugar and baking powder.
2. Combine oil, milk and egg in another bowl. Once done, add them all to the flour mixture.
3. Make sure that as your stir the mixture, blend them together until slightly lumpy.
4. In a hot greased griddle, pour-in at least ¼ cup of the batter to make each pancake.
5. To cook, ensure that the bottom is a bit brown, then turn and cook the other side, as well.

Nutrition:

Calories: 167;

Carbs: 50g;

Protein: 11g;

Fats: 11g;

Phosphorus: 176mg;

Potassium: 215mg;

Sodium: 70mg

## 160. Pasta with Indian Lentils

**Preparation Time:** 5 minutes
**Cooking Time:** 0 minutes
**Servings:** 6

**Ingredients:**

- ¼-½ cup fresh cilantro (chopped)
- 3 cups water
- 2 small dry red peppers (whole)
- 1 teaspoon turmeric
- 1 teaspoon ground cumin
- 2-3 cloves garlic (minced)
- 1 can (15 ounces) cubed Red bell peppers (with juice)
- 1 large onion (chopped)
- ½ cup dry lentils (rinsed)
- ½ cup orzo or tiny pasta

**Directions:**

1. In a skillet, combine all ingredients except for the cilantro then boil on medium-high heat.
2. Ensure to cover and slightly reduce heat to medium-low and simmer until pasta is tender for about 35 minutes.
3. Afterwards, take out the chili peppers then add cilantro and top it with low-fat sour cream.

**Nutrition:**

Calories: 175;

Carbs: 40g;

Protein: 3g;

Fats: 2g;

Phosphorus: 139mg;

Potassium: 513mg;

Sodium: 61mg

## 161. Shrimp Bruschetta

**Preparation Time:** 15 minutes

**Cooking Time:** 10 minutes

**Servings:** 4

**Ingredients:**
- 13 oz. shrimps, peeled
- 1 tablespoon tomato sauce
- ½ teaspoon Splenda
- ¼ teaspoon garlic powder
- 1 teaspoon fresh parsley, chopped
- ½ teaspoon olive oil
- 1 teaspoon lemon juice
- 4 whole-grain bread slices
- 1 cup water, for cooking

**Directions:**
1. In the saucepan, pour water and bring it to boil.
2. Add shrimps and boil them over the high heat for 5 minutes.
3. After this, drain shrimps and chill them to the room temperature.
4. Mix up together shrimps with Splenda, garlic powder, tomato sauce, and fresh parsley.
5. Add lemon juice and stir gently.
6. Preheat the oven to 360f.
7. Coat the slice of bread with olive oil and bake for 3 minutes.
8. Then place the shrimp mixture on the bread. Bruschetta is cooked.

**Nutrition:**

Calories 199,

Fat 3.7,

Fiber 2.1,

Carbs 15.3,

Protein 24.1

Calcium 79mg,

Phosphorous 316mg,

Potassium 227mg

Sodium: 121 mg

## 162. Strawberry Muesli

**Preparation Time:** 10 minutes

**Cooking Time:** 30 minutes

**Servings:** 4

**Ingredients:**
- 2 cups Greek yogurt
- 1 ½ cup strawberries, sliced
- 1 ½ cup Muesli
- 4 teaspoon maple syrup
- ¾ teaspoon ground cinnamon

**Directions:**
1. Put Greek yogurt in the food processor.
2. Add 1 cup of strawberries, maple syrup, and ground cinnamon.
3. Blend the ingredients until you get smooth mass.
4. Transfer the yogurt mass in the serving bowls.
5. Add Muesli and stir well.
6. Leave the meal for 30 minutes in the fridge.
7. After this, decorate it with remaining sliced strawberries.

**Nutrition:**

Calories 149,

Fat 2.6,

Fiber 3.6,

Carbs 21.6,

Protein 12

Calcium 69mg,

Phosphorous 216mg,

Potassium 227mg

Sodium: 151 mg

## 163. Yogurt Bulgur

**Preparation Time:** 10 minutes
**Cooking Time:** 15 minutes
**Servings:** 3
**Ingredients:**
- 1 cup bulgur
- 2 cups Greek yogurt
- 1 ½ cup water
- ½ teaspoon salt
- 1 teaspoon olive oil

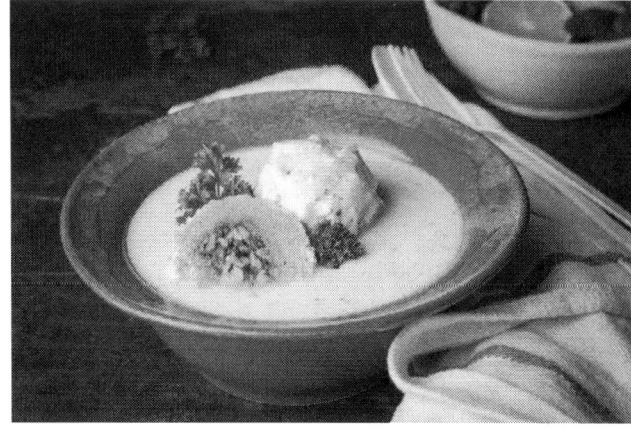

**Directions:**
1. Pour olive oil in the saucepan and add bulgur.
2. Roast it over the medium heat for 2-3 minutes. Stir it from time to time.
3. After this, add salt and water.
4. Close the lid and cook bulgur for 15 minutes over the medium heat.
5. Then chill the cooked bulgur well and combine it with Greek yogurt. Stir it carefully.
6. Transfer the cooked meal into the serving plates. The yogurt bulgur tastes the best when it is cold.

**Nutrition:**
Calories 274,
Fat 4.9,
Fiber 8.5,
Carbs 40.8,
Protein 19.2
Calcium 39mg,
Phosphorous 216mg,
Potassium 237mg
Sodium: 131 mg

## 164. Mozzarella Cheese Omelet

**Preparation Time:** 10 minutes

**Cooking Time:** 5 minutes

**Servings:** 1

**Ingredients:**

- 4 eggs, beaten
- 1/4 cup mozzarella cheese, shredded
- 4 tomato slices
- 1/4 tsp. Italian seasoning
- 1/4 tsp. dried oregano
- Pepper
- Salt

**Directions:**

1. In a small bowl, whisk eggs with salt.
2. Spray pan with cooking spray and heat over medium heat.
3. Pour egg mixture into the pan and cook over medium heat.
4. Once eggs are set then sprinkle oregano and Italian seasoning on top.
5. Arrange tomato slices on top of the omelet and sprinkle with shredded cheese.
6. Cook omelet for 1 minute.
7. Serve and enjoy.

**Nutrition:**

Calories 285

Fat 19g

Carbohydrates 4g

Sugar 3g

Protein 25g

Cholesterol 655 mg

# CHAPTER 10:

# Lunch

### 165. Couscous and Sherry Vinaigrette

**Preparation Time:** 10 minutes

**Cooking Time:** 30 minutes

**Servings:** 6

**Ingredients:**

For Sherry Vinaigrette: (makes 2/3 cup)

- 2 tablespoons sherry vinegar - ¼ cup lemon juice
- 1 clove garlic, pressed - 1/3 cup olive oil

**For Roasted Carrots, Cranberries and Couscous:**

- 1 medium onion, sliced
- 2 large carrots, sliced - 2 tablespoons extra-virgin olive oil
- 2 cups pearl couscous - 2 ½ to 3 cups no sodium vegetable broth
- ½ cup dried cranberries - ¼ cup Sherry vinaigrette

**Directions:**

**For Sherry Vinaigrette:**

1. Beat the vinegar with garlic and lemon juice.
2. Slowly whisk in olive oil. - Store refrigerated in a glass jar.

**For Carrots, Cranberries and Couscous:**

1. Preheat oven to 400°F. Spray a baking dish with cooking spray (olive oil) and place the carrots and onions on it. Roast the vegetables in oven for about 20 minutes until starting to brown. Stir halfway cooking. Heat the couscous in a pan over medium-high heat. Toast the couscous until light brown (about 10 minutes). Stir well. Check the package instructions for the amount of liquid needed for couscous.
2. Bring to a boil the added vegetable stock. Cover and reduce for about 10 minutes. The vegetable stock has to be absorbed. In a mixing bowl, incorporate the couscous with the onions, carrots, cranberries, and sherry vinaigrette. Serve and enjoy!

**Nutrition:**

Calories 365 Fat 11 g Cholesterol 0 mg Carbohydrate 58 g Sugar 11 g Fiber 4 g
Protein 9 g Sodium 95 mg Calcium 41 mg Phosphorus 119 mg Potassium 264 mg

## 166. Persian Chicken

**Preparation Time:** 10 minutes,
**Cooking Time:** 20 minutes
**Servings:** 6
**Ingredients:**

- 1/2 small sweet onion,
- 1/4 cup freshly squeezed lemon juice
- 1 tablespoon dried oregano
- 1/2 tablespoon of sweet paprika,
- 1/2 tablespoon of ground cumin
- 1/2 cup olive oil
- 6 boneless, skinless chicken thighs

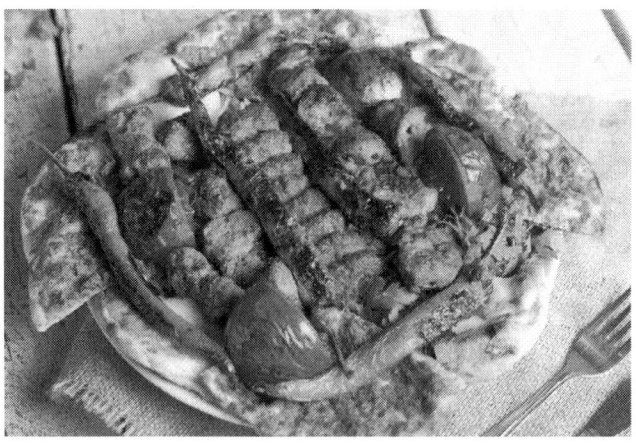

**Directions:**

1. Put the vegetables in a blender. Mix it well.
2. Put the olive while the motor is running.
3. In a sealable bag for the freezer, place the chicken thighs and put the mixture in the sealable bag.
4. Refrigerate it for 2 hours, while turning it two times.
5. Remove the marinade thighs and discard the additional marinade. Preheat to medium the barbecue. Grill the chicken, turning once or until the internal

**Nutrition:** Fat: 21 g; Carbohydrates: 3 g; Potassium: 220 mg; Sodium: 86 mg; Protein: 22 g

## 167. Ratatouille

**Preparation Time:** 5 minutes
**Cooking Time:** 15 minutes
**Servings:** 4
**Ingredients:**

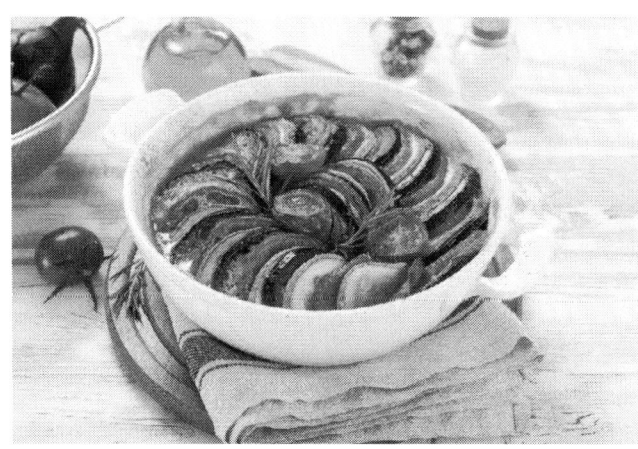

- 1 cup Water
- 3 tbsp. oil
- 2 Zucchinis, sliced in rings
- 2 Eggplants, sliced in rings
- 1 medium Red Onion, sliced in thin rings
- 3 cloves Garlic, minced
- 2 sprigs Fresh Thyme
- Salt to taste
- Black Pepper to taste
- 4 tsp Plain Vinegar

**Directions:**

1. Place all veggies in a bowl, sprinkle with salt and pepper; toss. Line foil in a spring form tin and arrange 1 slice each of the vegetables in, one after the other in a tight circular arrangement.
2. Fill the entire tin. Sprinkle the garlic over, some more black pepper and salt, and arrange the thyme sprigs on top. Drizzle olive oil and vinegar over the veggies.
3. Place a trivet to fit in the Instant Pot, pour the water in and place the veggies on the trivet. Seal the lid, secure the pressure valve and select Manual mode on High Pressure for 6 minutes. Once ready, quickly release the pressure. Carefully remove the tin and serve ratatouille.

**Nutrition:** Calories 152, Protein 2g, Net Carbs 4g, Fat 12g

## 168. Jicama Noodles

**Preparation Time:** 15 minutes

**Cooking Time:** 7 minutes

**Servings:** 6

**Ingredients:**

- 1-pound jicama, peeled
- 2 tablespoons butter
- 1 teaspoon chili flakes
- 1 teaspoon salt
- ¾ cup of water

**Directions:**

1. Spiralize jicama with the help of spiralizer and place in jicama spirals in the saucepan.
2. Add butter, chili flakes, and salt.
3. Then add water and preheat the ingredients until the butter is melted.
4. Mix up it well.
5. Close the lid and cook noodles for 4 minutes over the medium heat.
6. Stir the jicama noodles well before transferring them in the serving plates.

**Nutrition:**

Calories 63,

Fat 3.9,

Fiber 3.7,

Carbs 6.7,

Protein 0.6

## 169. Crack Slaw

**Preparation Time:** 15 minutes

**Cooking Time:** 10 minutes

**Servings:** 6

**Ingredients:**
- 1 cup cauliflower rice
- 1 tablespoon sriracha
- 1 teaspoon tahini paste
- 1 teaspoon sesame seeds
- 1 tablespoon lemon juice
- 1 teaspoon olive oil
- 1 teaspoon butter
- ½ teaspoon salt
- 2 cups coleslaw

**Directions:**
1. Toss the butter in the skillet and melt it.
2. Add cauliflower rice and sprinkle it with sriracha and tahini paste.
3. Mix up the vegetables and cook them for 10 minutes over the medium heat. Stir them from time to time.
4. When the cauliflower is cooked, transfer it into the big plate.
5. Add coleslaw and stir gently.
6. Then sprinkle the salad with sesame seeds, lemon juice, olive oil, and salt.
7. Mix up well.

**Nutrition:**

Calories 76,

Fat 5.8,

Fiber 0.6,

Carbs 6,

Protein 1.1

## 170. Vegan Chili

**Preparation Time:** 10 minutes
**Cooking Time:** 20 minutes
**Servings:** 4

**Ingredients:**

- 1 cup cremini mushrooms, chopped
- 1 zucchini, chopped
- 1 bell pepper, diced
- 1/3 cup crushed Red bell peppers
- 1 oz. celery stalk, chopped
- 1 teaspoon chili powder
- 1 teaspoon salt
- ½ teaspoon chili flakes
- ½ cup of water
- 1 tablespoon olive oil
- ½ teaspoon diced garlic
- ½ teaspoon ground black pepper
- 1 teaspoon of cocoa powder
- 2 oz. Cheddar cheese, grated

**Directions:**

1. Pour olive oil in the pan and preheat it.
2. Add chopped mushrooms and roast them for 5 minutes. Stir them from time to time.
3. After this, add chopped zucchini and bell pepper.
4. Sprinkle the vegetables with the chili powder, salt, chili flakes, diced garlic, and ground black pepper.
5. Stir the vegetables and cook them for 5 minutes more.
6. After this, add crushed Red bell peppers. Mix up well.
7. Bring the mixture to boil and add water and cocoa powder.
8. Then add celery stalk.
9. Mix up the chili well and close the lid.
10. Cook the chili for 10 minutes over the medium-low heat.
11. Then transfer the cooked vegan chili in the bowls and top with the grated cheese.

**Nutrition:**

Calories 123, Fat 8.6, Fiber 2.3, Carbs 7.6, Protein 5.6  Chow Mein

## 171. Chow Mein

**Preparation Time:** 10 minutes
**Cooking Time:** 10 minutes
**Servings:** 6

**Ingredients:**
- 7 oz. kelp noodles
- 5 oz. broccoli florets
- 1 tablespoon tahini sauce
- ¼ teaspoon minced ginger
- 1 teaspoon Sriracha
- ½ teaspoon garlic powder
- 1 cup of water

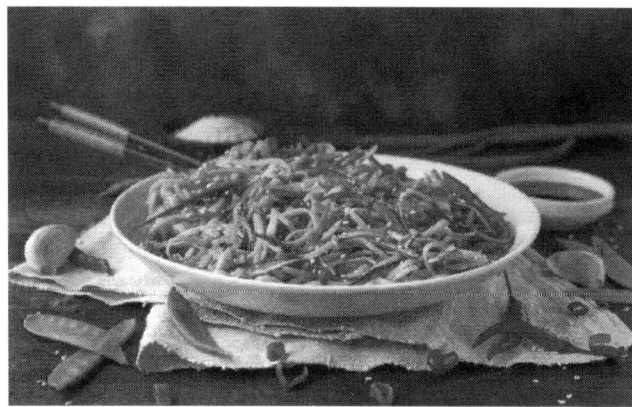

**Directions:**
1. Boil water in a sauce pan.
2. Add broccoli and boil for 4 minutes over the high heat.
3. Then drain water into the bowl and chill it tills the room temperature.
4. Soak the kelp noodles in the "broccoli water".
5. Meanwhile, place tahini sauce, sriracha, minced ginger, and garlic in the saucepan.
6. Bring the mixture to boil. Add oil if needed.
7. Then add broccoli and soaked noodles.
8. Add 3 tablespoons of "broccoli water".
9. Mix up the noodles and bring to boil.
10. Switch off the heat and transfer chow Mein in the serving bowls.

**Nutrition:**

Calories 18,

Fat 0.8,

Fiber 0.7,

Carbs 2.8,

Protein 0.9

## 172. Mushroom Tacos

**Preparation Time:** 10 minutes

**Cooking Time:** 15 minutes

**Servings:** 6

**Ingredients:**

- 6 collard greens leave
- 2 cups mushrooms, chopped
- 1 white onion, diced
- 1 tablespoon Taco seasoning
- 1 tablespoon coconut oil
- ½ teaspoon salt
- ¼ cup fresh parsley
- 1 tablespoon mayonnaise

**Directions:**

1. Put the coconut oil in the skillet and melt it.
2. Add chopped mushrooms and diced onion. Mix up the ingredients.
3. Close the lid and cook them for 10 minutes.
4. After this, sprinkle the vegetables with Taco seasoning, salt, and add fresh parsley.
5. Mix up the mixture and cook for 5 minutes more.
6. Then add mayonnaise and stir well.
7. Chill the mushroom mixture little.
8. Fill the collard green leaves with the mushroom mixture and fold up them.

**Nutrition:**

Calories 52,

Fat 3.3,

Fiber 1.2,

Carbs 5.1,

Protein 1.4

## 173. Lime Green lettuce and Chickpeas Salad

**Preparation Time:** 10 minutes

**Cooking Time:** 0 minutes

**Servings:** 4

**Ingredients:**

- 16 ounces canned chickpeas, drained and rinsed
- 2 cups baby green lettuce leaves
- ½ tablespoon lime juice
- 2 tablespoons olive oil
- 1 teaspoon cumin, ground
- Sea salt and black pepper
- ½ teaspoon chili flakes

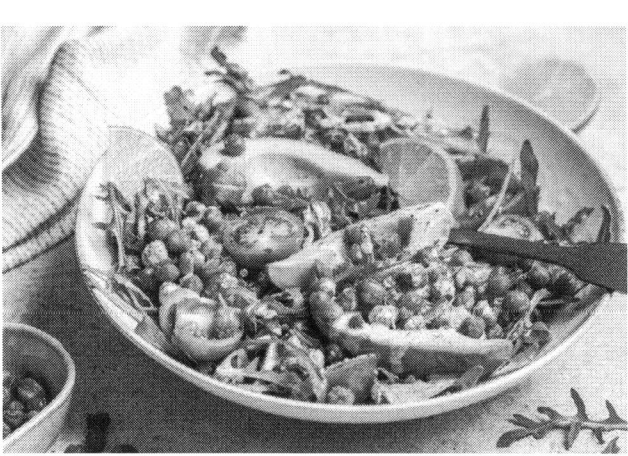

**Directions:**

1. In a bowl, mix the chickpeas with the green lettuce and the rest of the ingredients, toss and serve cold.

**Nutrition:**

Calories 240,

Fat 8.2,

Fiber 5.3,

Carbs 11.6,

Protein 12

## 174. Fried Rice with Kale

**Preparation Time:** 10 minutes
**Cooking Time:** 12 minutes
**Servings:** 4

**Ingredients:**

- 2 tbsp. Extra virgin oil
- 8 oz. Tofu, chopped
- 6 Scallion, white and green parts, thinly sliced
- 2 cups Kale, stemmed and chopped
- 3 cups Cooked white rice
- ¼ cup Stir fry sauce

**Directions:**

1. In a huge skillet on medium-high heat, warm the oil until it shimmers.
2. Add the tofu, scallions, and kale. Cook for 5 to 7 minutes, frequently stirring, until the vegetables are soft.
3. Add the white rice and stir-fry sauce. Cook for 3 to 5 minutes, occasionally stirring, until heated through.

**Nutrition:**

Calories: 301
Total Fat: 11g
Total Carbs: 36g
Sugar: 1g
Fiber: 3g
Protein: 16g
Sodium: 2,535mg

## 175. Stir-Fried Gingery Veggies

**Preparation Time:** 10 minutes
**Cooking Time:** 10 minutes
**Servings:** 4

**Ingredients:**
- 1 tablespoon oil
- 3 cloves of garlic, minced
- 1 onion, chopped
- 1 thumb-size ginger, sliced
- 1 tablespoon water
- 1 large carrots, peeled and julienned and seedless
- 1 large green bell pepper, julienned and seedless
- 1 large yellow bell pepper, julienned and seedless
- 1 large red bell pepper, julienned and seedless
- 1 zucchini, julienned
- Salt and pepper to taste

**Directions:**
1. Heat oil in a nonstick saucepan over a high flame and sauté the garlic, onion, and ginger until fragrant.
2. Stir in the rest of the ingredients.
3. Keep on stirring for at least 5 minutes until vegetables are tender.
4. Serve and enjoy.

**Nutrition:**
Calories 70
Total Fat 4g
Saturated Fat 1g
Total Carbs 9g
Net Carbs 7g
Protein 1g
Sugar: 4g
Fiber 2g
Sodium 173mg
Potassium 163mg

# CHAPTER 11:

# Dinner

## 176. Fish En' Papillote

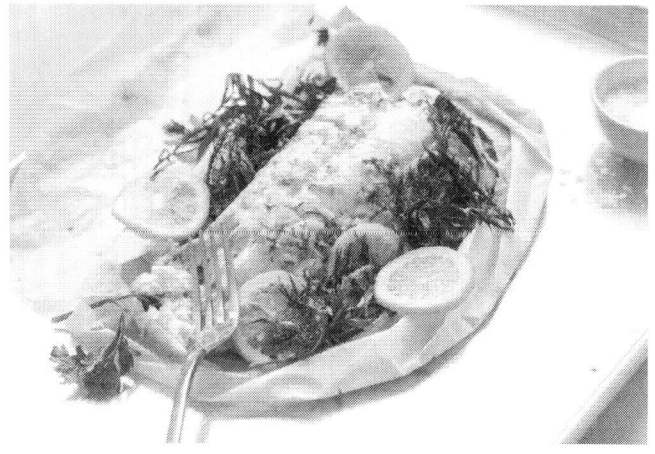

**Preparation Time:** 15 minutes

**Cooking Time:** 20 minutes

**Servings:** 3

**Ingredients:**
- 10 oz. snapper fillet
- 1 tablespoon fresh dill, chopped
- 1 white onion, peeled, sliced
- ½ teaspoon tarragon
- 1 tablespoon olive oil
- 1 teaspoon salt
- ½ teaspoon hot pepper
- 2 tablespoons sour cream

**Directions:**
1. Make the medium size packets from parchment and arrange them in the baking tray. Cut the snapper fillet into 3 and sprinkle them with salt, tarragon, and hot pepper.
2. Put the fish fillets in the parchment packets. Then top the fish with olive oil, sour cream, sliced onion, and fresh dill. Bake the fish for 20 minutes at 355F. Serve.

**Nutrition:**

Calories 204

Fat 8.2g

Carbs 4.6g

Protein 27.2g

Phosphorus 138.8 mg

Potassium 181.9 mg

Sodium 59.6 mg

## 177. Pesto Pasta Salad

**Preparation Time:** 15 minutes
**Cooking Time:** 15 minutes
Servings: 4

**Ingredients:**
- 1 cup fresh basil leaves
- ½ cup packed fresh flat-leaf parsley leaves
- ½ cup arugula, chopped
- 2 tablespoons Parmesan cheese, grated
- ¼ cup extra-virgin olive oil
- 3 tablespoons mayonnaise
- 2 tablespoons water
- 12 ounces whole-wheat rotini pasta
- 1 red bell pepper, chopped
- 1 medium yellow summer squash, sliced
- 1 cup frozen baby peas

**Directions:**
1. Boil water in a large pot.
2. Meanwhile, combine the basil, parsley, arugula, cheese, and olive oil in a blender or food processor. Process until the herbs are finely chopped. Add the mayonnaise and water, then process again. Set aside.
3. Prepare the pasta to the pot of boiling water; cook according to package directions, about 8 to 9 minutes. Drain well, reserving ¼ cup of the cooking liquid.
4. Combine the pesto, pasta, bell pepper, squash, and peas in a large bowl and toss gently, adding enough reserved pasta cooking liquid to make a sauce on the salad. Serve immediately or cover and chill, then serve.
5. Store covered in the refrigerator for up to 3 days.

**Nutrition:**
Calories: 378
Fat: 24g
Carbohydrates: 35g
Protein: 9g
Sodium: 163mg
Potassium: 472mg
Phosphorus: 213mg

## 178. Barley Blueberry Salad

**Preparation Time: 15 minutes**

**Cooking Time: 15 minutes**

**Servings: 4**

**Ingredients:**
- 1 cup quick-cooking barley
- 3 cups low-sodium vegetable broth
- 3 tablespoons extra-virgin olive oil
- 2 tablespoons freshly squeezed lemon juice
- 1 teaspoon yellow mustard
- 1 teaspoon honey
- 2 cups blueberries
- ¼ cup crumbled feta cheese

**Directions:**
1. Combine the barley and vegetable broth in a medium saucepan and bring to a simmer.
2. Reduce the heat to low, partially cover the pan, and simmer for 10 to 12 minutes or until the barley is tender.
3. Meanwhile, whisk together the olive oil, lemon juice, mustard, and honey in a serving bowl until blended.
4. Drain the barley if necessary and add to the bowl; toss to combine.
5. Add the blueberries, and feta and toss gently. Serve.

**Nutrition:**

Calories: 345

Fat 16g

Carbohydrates: 44g

Protein: 7g

Sodium: 259mg

Potassium: 301mg

Phosphorus: 152mg

## 179. Pasta with Creamy Broccoli Sauce

**Preparation Time:** 15 minutes

**Cooking Time:** 15 minutes

**Servings:** 4

**Ingredients:**

1. 2 tablespoons olive oil
2. 1-pound broccoli florets
3. 3 garlic cloves, halved
4. 1 cup low-sodium vegetable broth
5. ½ pound whole-wheat spaghetti pasta
6. 4 ounces cream cheese
7. 1 teaspoon dried basil leaves
8. ½ cup grated Parmesan cheese

**Directions:**

1. Prepare a large pot of water to a boil.
2. Put olive oil in a large skillet. Sauté the broccoli and garlic for 3 minutes.
3. Add the broth to the skillet and bring to a simmer. Reduce the heat to low, partially cover the skillet, and simmer until the broccoli is tender about 5 to 6 minutes.
4. Cook the pasta according to package directions. Drain when al dente, reserving 1 cup pasta water.
5. When the broccoli is tender, add the cream cheese and basil—purée using an immersion blender.
6. Put mixture into a food processor, about half at a time, and purée until smooth and transfer the sauce back into the skillet.
7. Add the cooked pasta to the broccoli sauce. Toss, adding enough pasta water until the sauce coats the pasta completely. Sprinkle with the Parmesan and serve.

**Nutrition:**

Calories: 302

Fat 14g

Carbohydrates: 36g

Protein: 11g

Sodium: 260mg

Potassium: 375mg

Phosphorus: 223mg

## 180. Asparagus Fried Rice

**Preparation Time: 10 minutes**

**Cooking Time: 10 minutes**

**Servings: 1**

**Ingredients:**

- 3 large eggs, beaten
- ½ teaspoon ground ginger
- 2 teaspoons low-sodium soy sauce
- 2 tablespoons olive oil
- 1 onion, diced
- 4 garlic cloves, minced
- 1 cup sliced cremini mushrooms
- 1 (10-ounce) package frozen white rice, thawed
- 8 ounces fresh asparagus, about 15 spears, cut into 1-inch pieces
- 1 teaspoon sesame oil

**Directions:**

1. Whisk the eggs, ginger, and soy sauce in a small bowl and set aside.
2. Heat the olive oil in a medium skillet or wok over medium heat.
3. Add the onion and garlic and sauté for 2 minutes until tender crisp.
4. Add the mushrooms and rice; stir-fry for 3 minutes longer.
5. Put asparagus and cook for 2 minutes.6.
6. Pour in the egg mixture. Stir the eggs until cooked through, 2 to 3 minutes, and stir into the rice mixture.
7. Sprinkle the fried rice with the sesame oil and serve.

**Nutrition:**

Calories: 247

Fat: 13g

Carbohydrates: 25g

Protein: 9g

Sodium: 149mg

Potassium: 367mg

Phosphorus: 206mg

## 181. Beef and Chili Stew

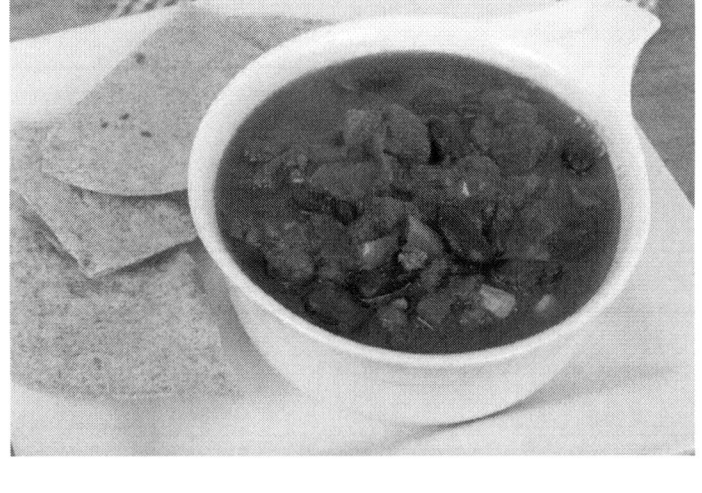

**Preparation Time:** 15 minutes

**Cooking Time:** 7 hours

**Servings:** 6

**Ingredients:**

- 1/2 medium red onion, sliced thinly
- 1/2 tablespoon vegetable oil
- 10ounce of flat-cut beef brisket, whole
- ½ cup low sodium stock
- ¾ cup of water
- ½ tablespoon honey
- ½ tablespoon chili powder
- ½ teaspoon smoked paprika
- ½ teaspoon dried thyme
- 1 teaspoon black pepper
- 1 tablespoon corn starch

**Directions:**

1. Throw the sliced onion into the slow cooker first. Add a splash of oil to a large hot skillet and briefly seal the beef on all sides.
2. Remove the beef, then place it in the slow cooker. Add the stock, water, honey, and spices to the same skillet you cooked the beef meat.
3. Allow the juice to simmer until the volume is reduced by about half. Pour the juice over beef in the slow cooker. Cook on low within 7 hours.
4. Transfer the beef to your platter, shred it using two forks. Put the rest of the juice into a medium saucepan. Bring it to a simmer.
5. Whisk the cornstarch with two tablespoons of water. Add to the juice and cook until slightly thickened.
6. For a thicker sauce, simmer and reduce the juice a bit more before adding cornstarch. Put the sauce on the meat and serve.

**Nutrition:**

Calories: 128 Protein: 13g

Carbohydrates: 6g Fat: 6g

Sodium: 228mg Potassium: 202mg

Phosphorus: 119mg

## 182. Sticky Pulled Beef Open Sandwiches

**Preparation Time:** 15 minutes

**Cooking Time:** 5 hours

**Servings:** 5

**Ingredients:**

- ½ cup of green onion, sliced
- 2 garlic cloves
- 2 tablespoons of fresh parsley
- 2 large carrots
- 7ounce of flat-cut beef brisket, whole
- 1 tablespoon of smoked paprika
- 1 teaspoon dried parsley
- 1 teaspoon of brown sugar
- ½ teaspoon of black pepper
- 2 tablespoon of olive oil
- ¼ cup of red wine
- 8 tablespoon of cider vinegar
- 3 cups of water
- 5 slices white bread
- 1 cup of arugula to garnish

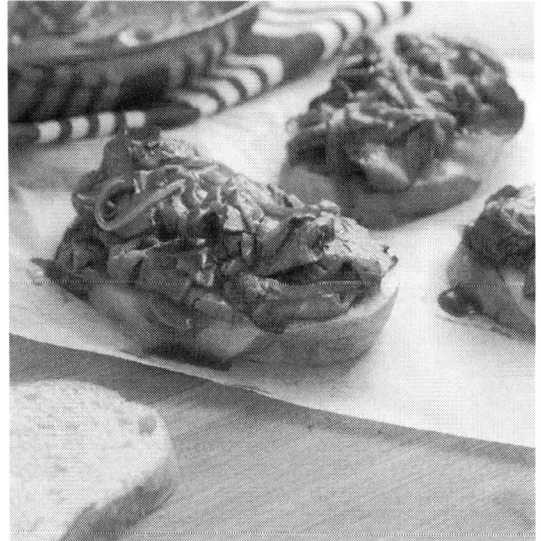

**Directions:**

1. Finely chop the green onion, garlic, and fresh parsley. Grate the carrot. Put the beef in to roast in a slow cooker.
2. Add the chopped onion, garlic, and remaining ingredients, leaving the rolls, fresh parsley, and arugula to one side. Stir in the slow cooker to combine.
3. Cover and cook on low within 8 1/2 to 10 hours or on high for 4 to 5 hours until tender. Remove the meat from the slow cooker. Shred the meat using two forks.
4. Return the meat to the broth to keep it warm until ready to serve. Lightly toast the bread and top with shredded beef, arugula, fresh parsley, and ½ spoon of the broth. Serve.

**Nutrition:**

Calories: 273 Protein: 15g Carbohydrates: 20g

Fat: 11g Sodium: 308mg Potassium: 399mg Phosphorus: 159mg

## 183. Herby Beef Stroganoff and Fluffy Rice

**Preparation Time:** 15 minutes

**Cooking Time:** 5 hours

**Servings:** 6

**Ingredients:**

- ½ cup onion
- 2 garlic cloves
- 9ounce of flat-cut beef brisket, cut into 1" cubes
- ½ cup of reduced-sodium beef stock
- 1/3 cup red wine
- ½ teaspoon dried oregano
- ¼ teaspoon freshly ground black pepper
- ½ teaspoon dried thyme
- ½ teaspoon of saffron
- ½ cup almond milk (unenriched)
- ¼ cup all-purpose flour
- 1 cup of water
- 2 ½ cups of white rice

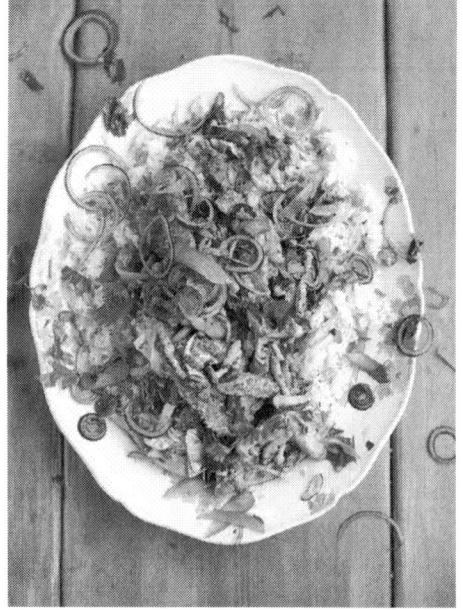

**Directions:**

1. Dice the onion, then mince the garlic cloves. Mix the beef, stock, wine, onion, garlic, oregano, pepper, thyme, and saffron in your slow cooker.
2. Cover and cook on high within 4-5 hours. Combine the almond milk, flour, and water. Whisk together until smooth.
3. Add the flour mixture to the slow cooker. Cook for another 15 to 25 minutes until the stroganoff is thick.
4. Cook the rice using the package instructions, leaving out the salt. Drain off the excess water. Serve the stroganoff over the rice.

**Nutrition:**

Calories: 241

Protein: 15g

Carbohydrates: 29g

Fat: 5g

Sodium: 182mg

Potassium: 206mg

Phosphorus: 151mg

## 184. Chunky Beef and Potato Slow Roast

**Preparation Time:** 15 minutes

**Cooking Time:** 5-6 hours

**Servings:** 12

**Ingredients:**

- 3 cups of peeled potatoes, chunked
- 1 cup of onion
- 2 garlic cloves, chopped
- 1 ¼ pound flat-cut beef brisket, fat trimmed
- 2 cups of water
- 1 teaspoon of chili powder
- 1 tablespoon of dried rosemary

For the sauce:

- 1 tablespoon of freshly grated horseradish
- ½ cup of almond milk (unenriched)
- 1 tablespoon lemon juice (freshly squeezed)
- 1 garlic clove, minced
- A pinch of cayenne pepper

**Directions:**

1. Double boil the potatoes to reduce their potassium content. Chop the onion and the garlic. Place the beef brisket in a slow cooker. Combine water, chopped garlic, chili powder, and rosemary.
2. Pour the mixture over the brisket. Cover and cook on high within 4-5 hours until the meat is very tender. Drain the potatoes and add them to the slow cooker.
3. Adjust the heat to high and cook covered until the potatoes are tender. Prepare the horseradish sauce by whisking together horseradish, milk, lemon juice, minced garlic, and cayenne pepper.
4. Cover and refrigerate. Serve your casserole with a dash of horseradish sauce on the side.

**Nutrition:**

Calories: 199

Protein: 21g

Carbohydrates: 12g

Fat: 7g

Sodium: 282mg

Potassium: 317

Phosphorus: 191mg

## 185. Spiced Lamb Burgers

**Preparation Time:** 10 minutes
**Cooking Time:** 20 minutes
**Servings:** 2
**Ingredients:**

- 1 tablespoon extra-virgin olive oil
- 1 teaspoon cumin
- ½ finely diced red onion
- 1 minced garlic clove
- 1 teaspoon harissa spices
- 1 cup arugula
- 1 juiced lemon
- 6-ounce lean ground lamb
- 1 tablespoon parsley
- ½ cup low-fat plain yogurt

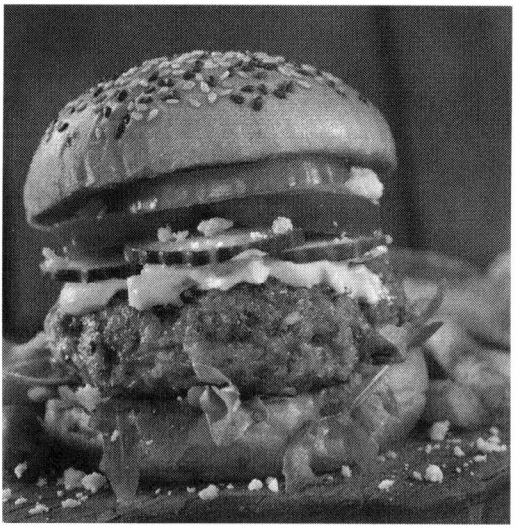

**Directions:**

1. Preheat the broiler on medium to high heat. Mix the ground lamb, red onion, parsley, Harissa spices, and olive oil until combined.
2. Shape 1-inch thick patties using wet hands. Add the patties to a baking tray and place under the broiler for 7-8 minutes on each side. Mix the yogurt, lemon juice, and cumin and serve over the lamb burgers with arugula's side salad.

**Nutrition:**

Calories 306

Fat 20g

Carbs 10g

Phosphorus 269mg

Potassium 492mg

Sodium 86mg

Protein 23g

## 186. Pork Loins with Leeks

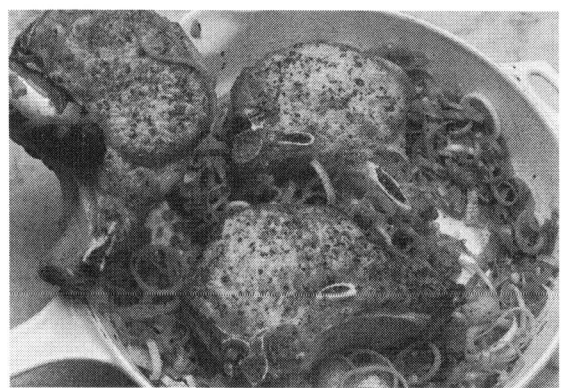

**Preparation Time:** 10 minutes
**Cooking Time:** 35 minutes
**Servings:** 2
**Ingredients:**
- 1 sliced leek
- 1 tablespoon mustard seeds
- 6-ounce pork tenderloin
- 1 tablespoon cumin seeds
- 1 tablespoon dry mustard
- 1 tablespoon extra-virgin oil

**Directions:**
1. Preheat the broiler to medium-high heat. In a dry skillet, heat mustard and cumin seeds until they start to pop (3-5 minutes). Grind seeds using a pestle and mortar or blender and then mix in the dry mustard.
2. Massage the pork on all sides using the mustard blend and add to a baking tray to broil for 25-30 minutes or until cooked through. Turn once halfway through.
3. Remove and place to one side, then heat-up the oil in a pan on medium heat and add the leeks for 5-6 minutes or until soft. Serve the pork tenderloin on a bed of leeks and enjoy it!

**Nutrition:**
Calories 139
Fat 5g
Carbs 2g
Phosphorus 278mg
Potassium 45mg
Sodium 47mg
Protein 18g

## 187. The Kale and Green lettuce Soup

**Preparation Time:** 5 minutes
**Cooking Time:** 10 minutes
**Servings:** 4
**Ingredients:**

- 3 ounces coconut oil
- 8 ounces kale, chopped
- 4 1/3 cups coconut almond milk
- Sunflower seeds and pepper to taste

**Directions:**

1. Take a skillet and place it over medium heat.
2. Add kale and sauté for 2-3 minutes
3. Add kale to blender.
4. Add water, spices, coconut almond milk to blender as well.
5. Blend until smooth and pour mix into bowl.
6. Serve and enjoy!

**Nutrition:** Calories: 124 Fat: 13g Carbohydrates: 7g Protein: 4.2g Phosphorus: 110mg Potassium: 117mg Sodium: 105mg

## 188. Japanese Onion Soup

**Preparation Time:** 15 minutes
**Cooking Time:** 45 minutes
**Servings:** 4
**Ingredients:**

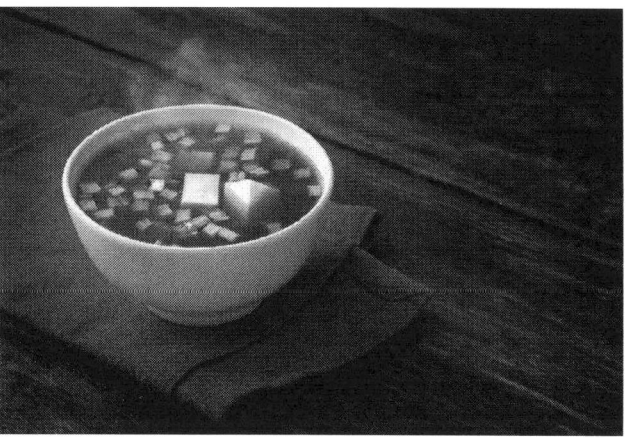

- ½ stalk celery, diced
- 1 small onion, diced
- ½ carrot, diced
- 1 teaspoon fresh ginger root, grated
- ¼ teaspoon fresh garlic, minced
- 2 tablespoons chicken stock
- 3 teaspoons beef bouillon granules
- 1 cup fresh shiitake, mushrooms
- 2 quarts water
- 1 cup baby Portobello mushrooms, sliced
- 1 tablespoon fresh chives

**Directions:**

1. Take a saucepan and place it over high heat, add water, bring to a boil.
2. Add beef bouillon, celery, onion, chicken stock, and carrots, half of the mushrooms, ginger, and garlic.
3. Put on the lid and reduce heat to medium, cook for 45 minutes.
4. Take another saucepan and add another half of mushrooms.
5. Once the soup is cooked, strain the soup into the pot with uncooked mushrooms.
6. Garnish with chives and enjoy!

**Nutrition:** Calories: 25 Fat: 0.2g Carbohydrates: 5g Protein: 1.4g Phosphorus: 210mg Potassium: 217mg Sodium: 75mg

## 189. Amazing Broccoli and Cauliflower Soup

**Preparation Time:** 10 minutes

**Cooking Time:** 8 hours

**Servings:** 4

**Ingredients:**

- 3 cups broccoli florets
- 2 cups cauliflower florets
- 2 garlic cloves, minced
- ½ cup shallots, chopped
- 1 carrot, chopped
- 3 ½ cups low sodium veggie stick
- Pinch of pepper
- 1 cup fat-free milk
- 6 ounces low-fat cheddar, shredded
- 1 cup non-fat Greek yogurt

**Directions:**

1. Add broccoli, cauliflower, garlic, shallots, carrot, stock, and pepper to your Slow Cooker.
2. Stir well and place lid.
3. Cook on LOW for 8 hours.
4. Add milk and cheese.
5. Use an immersion blender to smooth the soup.
6. Add yogurt and blend once more.
7. Ladle into bowls and enjoy!

**Nutrition:** Calories: 218 Fat: 11g Carbohydrates: 15g Protein: 12g Phosphorus: 206mg Potassium: 147mg Sodium: 75mg

# CHAPTER 12:

# Snacks

## 190. Lemon Thins

**Preparation Time:** 15 minutes
**Cooking Time:** 8 to 10 minutes
**Servings:** 30 cookies
**Ingredients:**

- Cooking spray
- 1 1/4 cups whole wheat pastry flour
- 1/3 cup cornstarch
- 1 1/2 teaspoons baking powder
- ¾ cup sugar, divided
- 2 tablespoons butter, softened
- 2 tablespoons extra-virgin olive oil
- 1 large egg white - 3 teaspoons freshly grated lemon zest
- 1 1/2 teaspoons vanilla extract
- 4 tablespoons freshly squeezed lemon juice

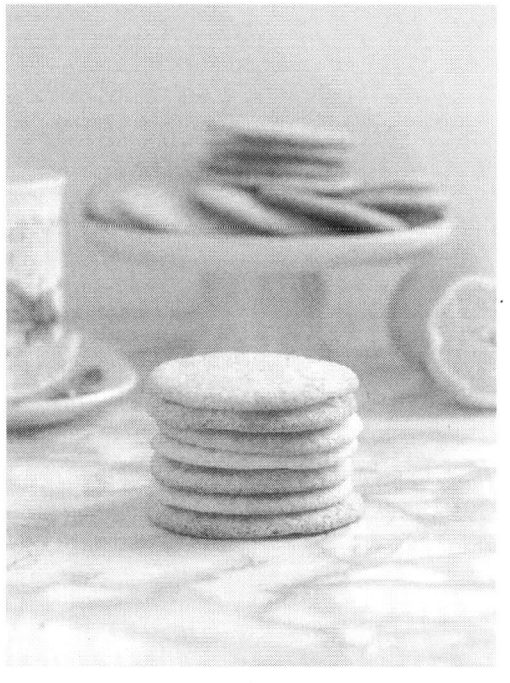

**Directions:**

1. Preheat the oven to 350°F. Coat two baking sheets with cooking spray.
2. In a mixing bowl, whisk together the flour, cornstarch, and baking powder.
3. In another mixing bowl beat 1/2 cup of the sugar, the butter, and olive oil with an electric mixer on medium speed until fluffy. Add the egg white, lemon zest, and vanilla and beat until smooth. Beat in the lemon juice. Add the dry ingredients to the wet ingredients and fold in with a rubber spatula just until combined. Drop the dough by the teaspoonful, 2 inches apart, onto the prepared baking sheets.
4. Place the remaining 1/4 cup sugar in a saucer. Coat the bottom of a wide-bottomed glass with cooking spray and dip it in the sugar. Flatten the dough with the glass bottom into 2 1/2-inch circles, dipping the glass in the sugar each time. Bake the cookies until they are just starting to brown around the edges, 8 to 10 minutes. Transfer to a flat surface (not a rack) to crisp.

**NUTRITION:** (1 cookie) Calories: 40; Total Fat 2g; Saturated Fat: 1g; Cholesterol: 2mg; Sodium: 26mg; Potassium: 3mg; Total Carbohydrate: 5g; Fiber: 1g; Protein: 1g

## 191. Snickerdoodle Chickpea Blondies

**Servings:** 15
**Preparation Time:** 10 minutes
**Cooking Time:** 30 to 35 minutes

**Ingredients:**

- 1 (15-ounce) can chickpeas, drained and rinsed
- 3 tablespoons nut butter of choice
- ¾ teaspoon baking powder
- 2 teaspoons vanilla extract
- 1/8 teaspoon baking soda
- ¾ cup brown sugar
- 1 tablespoon unsweetened applesauce
- 1/4 cup ground flaxseed meal
- 21/4 teaspoons cinnamon

**Directions:**

1. Preheat the oven to 350°F. Grease an 8-by-8-inch baking pan.
2. Blend all ingredients in a food processor until very smooth. Scoop into the prepared baking pan.
3. Bake until the tops are medium golden brown, 30 to 35 minutes. Allow the brownies to cool completely before cutting.

**NUTRITION:** Calories: 85; Total Fat 2g; Saturated Fat: 0g; Cholesterol: 0mg; Sodium: 7mg; Potassium: 62mg; Total Carbohydrate: 16g; Fiber: 2g; Protein: 3g

## 192. Chocolate Chia Seed Pudding

**Preparation Time:** 15 minutes, plus 3 to 5 hours or overnight to rest
**Cooking Time:** 0 minutes
**Servings:** 4

**Ingredients:**

- 1 1/2 cups unsweetened vanilla almond milk
- 1/4 cup unsweetened cocoa powder
- 1/4 cup maple syrup (or substitute any sweetener)
- 1/2 teaspoon vanilla extract
- 1/3 cup chia seeds
- 1/2 cup strawberries
- 1/4 cup blueberries
- 1/4 cup raspberries
- 2 tablespoons unsweetened coconut flakes
- 1/4 to 1/2 teaspoon ground cinnamon (optional)

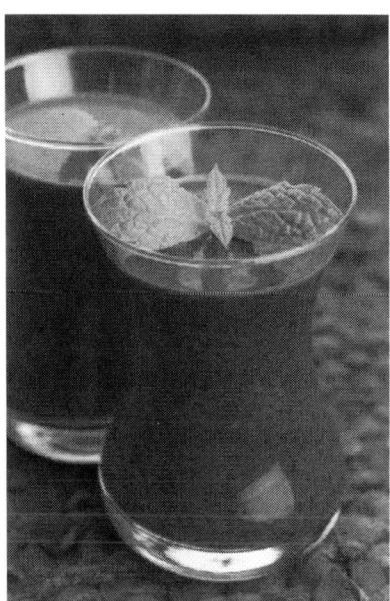

**Directions:**

1. Add the almond milk, cocoa powder, maple syrup, and vanilla extract to a blender and blend until smooth. Whisk in chia seeds.
2. In a small bowl, gently mash the strawberries with a fork. Distribute the strawberry mash evenly to the bottom of 4 glass jars.
3. Pour equal portions of the blended milk-cocoa mixture into each of the jars and let the pudding rest in the refrigerator until it achieves a pudding like consistency, at least 3 to 5 hours and up to overnight.

**NUTRITION:** Calories: 189; Total Fat 7g; Saturated Fat: 2g; Cholesterol: 0mg; Sodium: 60mg; Potassium: 232mg; Total Carbohydrate: 28g; Fiber: 10g; Protein: 6g

## 193. Chocolate-Mint Truffles

**Preparation Time:** 45 minutes

**Cooking Time:** 5 hours

**Servings:** 60 small truffles

**Ingredients:**

- 14 ounces semisweet chocolate, coarsely chopped
- ¾ cup half-and-half
- 1/2 teaspoon pure vanilla extract
- 11/2 teaspoon peppermint extract
- 2 tablespoons unsalted butter, softened
- ¾ cup naturally unsweetened or Dutch-process cocoa powder

**Directions:**

1. Place semisweet chocolate in a large heatproof bowl.
2. Microwave in four 15-second increments, stirring after each, for a total of 60 seconds. Stir until almost completely melted. Set aside.
3. In a small saucepan over medium heat, heat the half-and-half, whisking occasionally, until it just begins to boil. Remove from the heat, then whisk in the vanilla and peppermint extracts.
4. Pour the mixture over the chocolate and, using a wooden spoon, gently stir in one direction.
5. Once the chocolate and cream are smooth, stir in the butter until it is combined and melted.
6. Cover with plastic wrap pressed on the top of the mixture, and then let it sit at room temperature for 30 minutes.
7. After 30 minutes, place the mixture in the refrigerator until it is thick and can hold a ball shape, about 5 hours.
8. Line a large baking sheet with parchment paper or a use a silicone baking mat. Set aside.
9. Remove the mixture from the refrigerator. Place the cocoa powder in a bowl.
10. Scoop 1 teaspoon of the ganache and, using your hands, roll into a ball. Roll the ball in the cocoa powder, the place on the prepared baking sheet. (You can coat your palms with a little cocoa powder to prevent sticking).
11. Serve immediately or cover and store at room temperature for up to 1 week.

**NUTRITION:** Calories: 21; Total Fat 2g; Saturated Fat: 1g; Cholesterol: 2mg; Sodium: 2mg; Potassium: 21mg; Total Carbohydrate: 2g; Fiber: 1g; Protein: 0g

## 194. Personal Mango Pies

**Preparation Time:** 15 minutes
**Cooking Time:** 14 to 16 minutes
**Servings:** 12

**Ingredients:**
- Cooking spray
- 12 small wonton wrappers
- 1 tablespoon cornstarch
- 1/2 cup water
- 3 cups finely chopped mango (fresh, or thawed from frozen, no sugar added)
- 2 tablespoons brown sugar (not packed)
- 1/2 teaspoon cinnamon
- 1 tablespoon light whipped butter or buttery spread

**Directions:**
1. Unsweetened coconut flakes (optional)
2. Preheat the oven to 350°F.
3. Spray a 12-cup muffin pan with nonstick cooking spray.
4. Place a wonton wrapper into each cup of the muffin pan, pressing it into the bottom and up along the sides.
5. Lightly spray the wrappers with nonstick spray. Bake until lightly browned, about 8 minutes.
6. Meanwhile, in a medium nonstick saucepan, combine the cornstarch with the water and stir to dissolve. Add the mango, brown sugar, and cinnamon and turn heat to medium.
7. Stirring frequently, cook until the mangoes have slightly softened and the mixture is thick and gooey, 6 to 8 minutes.
8. Remove the mango mixture from heat and stir in the butter.
9. Spoon the mango mixture into wonton cups, about 3 tablespoons each. Top with coconut flakes (if using) and serve warm.

**NUTRITION:**
Calories: 61; Total Fat 1g; Saturated Fat: 0g; Cholesterol: 2mg; Sodium: 52mg; Potassium: 77mg; Total Carbohydrate: 14g; Fiber: 1g; Protein: 1g

## 195. Grilled Peach Sundaes

**Preparation Time:** 15 minutes

**Cooking Time:** 5 minutes

**Servings:** 1

**Ingredients:**

- 1 tbsp. toasted unsweetened coconut
- 1 tsp. canola oil
- 2 peaches, halved and pitted
- 2 scoops non-fat vanilla yogurt, frozen

**Directions:**

1. Brush the peaches with oil and grill until tender.
2. Place peach halves on a bowl and top with frozen yogurt and coconut.

**Nutrition:**

Calories: 61; carbs: 2g; protein: 2g; fats: 6g; phosphorus: 32mg; potassium: 85mg; sodium: 30mg

## 196. Blueberry Swirl Cake

**Preparation Time:** 15 minutes
**Cooking Time:** 45 minutes
**Servings:** 9
**Ingredients:**

- 1/2 cup margarine
- 1 1/4 cups reduced fat milk
- 1 cup granulated sugar
- 1 egg
- 1 egg white
- 1 tbsp. lemon zest, grated
- 1 tsp. cinnamon
- 1/3 cup light brown sugar
- 2 1/2 cups fresh blueberries
- 2 1/2 cups self-rising flour

**Directions:**

1. Cream the margarine and granulated sugar using an electric mixer at high speed until fluffy.
2. Add the egg and egg white and beat for another two minutes.
3. Add the lemon zest and reduce the speed to low.
4. Add the flour with milk alternately.
5. In a greased 13x19 pan, spread half of the batter and sprinkle with blueberry on top. Add the remaining batter.
6. Bake in a 350-degree Fahrenheit preheated oven for 45 minutes.
7. Let it cool on a wire rack before slicing and serving.

**Nutrition:**
Calories: 384; carbs: 63g; protein: 7g; fats: 13g; phosphorus: 264mg; potassium: 158mg; sodium: 456mg

## 197. Peanut Butter Cookies

**Preparation Time:** 15 minutes

**Cooking Time:** 24 minutes

**Servings:** 24

**Ingredients:**

- 1/4 cup granulated sugar
- 1 cup unsalted peanut butter
- 1 tsp. baking soda
- 2 cups all-purpose flour
- 2 large eggs
- 2 tbsp. butter
- 2 tsp. pure vanilla extract
- 4 ounces softened cream cheese

**Directions:**

1. Line a cookie sheet with a non-stick liner. Set aside.
2. In a bowl, mix flour, sugar and baking soda. Set aside.
3. On a mixing bowl, combine the butter, cream cheese and peanut butter.
4. Mix on high speed until it forms a smooth consistency. Add the eggs and vanilla gradually while mixing until it forms a smooth consistency.
5. Add the almond flour mixture slowly and mix until well combined.
6. The dough is ready once it starts to stick together into a ball.
7. Scoop the dough using a 1 tablespoon cookie scoop and drop each cookie on the prepared cookie sheet.
8. Press the cookie with a fork and bake for 10 to 12 minutes at 350oF.

**Nutrition:**

Calories: 138; carbs: 12g; protein: 4g; fats: 9g; phosphorus: 60mg; potassium: 84mg; sodium: 31mg

## 198. Deliciously Good Scones

**Preparation Time:** 15 minutes

**Cooking Time:** 12 minutes

**Servings:** 10

**Ingredients:**

- 1/4 cup dried cranberries
- 1/4 cup sunflower seeds
- 1/2 teaspoon baking soda
- 1 large egg
- 2 cups all-purpose flour
- 2 tablespoon honey

**Directions:**

1. Preheat the oven to 3500F.
2. Grease a baking sheet. Set aside.
3. In a bowl, mix the salt, baking soda and flour. Add the dried fruits, nuts and seeds. Set aside.
4. In another bowl, mix the honey and eggs.
5. Add the wet ingredients to the dry ingredients. Use your hands to mix the dough.
6. Create 10 small round dough and place them on the baking sheet.
7. Bake for 12 minutes.

**Nutrition:**

Calories: 44; carbs: 27g; protein: 4g; fats: 3g; phosphorus: 59mg; potassium: 92mg; sodium: 65mg

## 199. Mixed Berry Cobbler

**Preparation Time:** 15 minutes
**Cooking Time:** 4 hours
**Servings:** 8
**Ingredients:**

- 1/4 cup coconut milk
- 1/4 cup ghee
- 1/4 cup honey
- 1/2 cup almond flour
- 1/2 cup tapioca starch
- 1/2 tablespoon cinnamon
- 1/2 tablespoon coconut sugar
- 1 teaspoon vanilla
- 12 ounces frozen raspberries
- 16 ounces frozen wild blueberries
- 2 teaspoon baking powder
- 2 teaspoon tapioca starch

**Directions:**

1. Place the frozen berries in the slow cooker. Add honey and 2 teaspoons of tapioca starch. Mix to combine.
2. In a bowl, mix the tapioca starch, almond flour, coconut milk, ghee, baking powder and vanilla. Sweeten with sugar. Place this pastry mix on top of the berries.
3. Set the slow cooker for 4 hours.

**Nutrition:**

Calories: 146; carbs: 33g; protein: 1g; fats: 3g; phosphorus: 29mg; potassium: 133mg; sodium: 4mg

## 200. Blueberry Espresso Brownies

**Preparation Time:** 15 minutes
**Cooking Time:** 30 minutes
**Servings:** 12
**Ingredients:**

- 1/4 cup organic cocoa powder
- 1/4 teaspoon salt
- 1/2 cup raw honey
- 1/2 teaspoon baking soda
- 1 cup blueberries
- 1 cup coconut cream
- 1 tablespoon cinnamon
- 1 tablespoon ground coffee
- 2 teaspoon vanilla extract
- 3 eggs

**Directions:**

1. Preheat the oven to 3250F.
2. In a bow mix together coconut cream, honey, eggs, cinnamon, honey, vanilla, baking soda, coffee and salt.
3. Use a mixer to combine all ingredients.
4. Fold in the blueberries
5. Pour the batter in a greased baking dish and bake for 30 minutes or until a toothpick inserted in the middle comes out clean.
6. Remove from the oven and let it cool.

**Nutrition:**

Calories: 168; carbs: 20g; protein: 4g; fats: 10g; phosphorus: 79mg; potassium: 169mg; sodium: 129mg

## 201. Coffee Brownies

**Preparation Time:** 15 minutes

**Cooking Time:** 20 minutes

**Servings:** 4

**Ingredients:**

- 3 eggs, beaten
- 2 tablespoons cocoa powder
- 2 teaspoons Erythritol
- 1/2 cup almond flour
- 1/2 cup organic almond milk

**Directions:**

1. Place the eggs in the mixing bowl and combine them with Erythritol and almond milk.
2. With the help of the hand mixer, whisk the liquid until homogenous.
3. Then add almond flour and cocoa powder.
4. Whisk the mixture until smooth.
5. Take the non-sticky brownie mold and transfer the cocoa mass inside it.
6. Flatten it gently with the help of the spatula. The flattened mass should be thin.
7. Preheat the oven to 365F.
8. Transfer the brownie in the oven and bake it for 20 minutes.
9. Then chill the cooked brownies at least till the room temperature and cut into serving bars.

**Nutrition:** calories 78, fat 5.8, fiber 1.3, carbs 2.7, protein 5.5

# Conclusion

As for your well-being and health, it's a good idea to see your doctor as often as possible to make sure you don't have any preventable problems you don't need to have. The kidneys are your body's channel for toxins (as is the liver), cleaning the blood of unknown substances and toxins that are removed from things like preservatives in the food and other toxins. The moment you eat without control and fill your body with toxins, food, drink (liquor or alcohol, for example), or even the air you inhale in general, your body will also convert several things that appear to be benign until the body's organs convert them to things like formaldehyde, due to a synthetic response and transformation phase.

You likely had little knowledge about your kidneys before. You probably didn't know how you could take steps to improve your kidney health and decrease the risk of developing kidney failure. However, through reading this book, you now understand the power of the human kidney, as well as the prognosis of chronic kidney disease. While over thirty-million Americans are being affected by kidney disease, you can now take steps to be one of the people who is actively working to promote your kidney health.

These stats are alarming, which is why it is necessary to take proper care of your kidneys, starting with a kidney-friendly diet. These recipes are ideal whether you have been diagnosed with a kidney problem or you want to prevent any kidney issue. This isn't a condition that occurs without any forethought; it is a dynamic issue and in that it very well may be both found early and treated, diet changed, and settling what is causing the issue is conceivable. It's conceivable to have partial renal failure yet, as a rule; it requires some time (or downright poor diet for a short time) to arrive at absolute renal failure. You would prefer not to reach total renal failure since this will require standard dialysis treatments to save your life.

One such case is a large part of the dietary sugars used in diet sodas - for example, aspartame is converted to formaldehyde in the body. These toxins must be excreted or they can cause disease, renal (kidney) failure, malignant growth, and various other painful problems

Dialysis treatments explicitly clean the blood of waste and toxins in the blood utilizing a machine in light of the fact that your body can no longer carry out the responsibility. Without treatments, you could die a very painful death. Renal failure can be the consequence of long-haul diabetes, hypertension, unreliable diet, and can stem from other health concerns. A renal diet is tied in with directing the intake of protein and phosphorus in your eating routine. Restricting your sodium intake is likewise significant. By controlling these two variables you can control the vast majority of the toxins/waste made by your body, enabling your kidney to 100% function. In the event that you get this early enough and truly moderate your diets with extraordinary consideration, you could avert complete renal failure. If you get this early, you can take out the issue completely.

Printed in Great Britain
by Amazon